An Illustrated Guide to
The Knee

An Illustrated Guide to
The Knee

ALFRED J. TRIA, JR., M.D.
Associate Clinical Professor
Division of Orthopaedic Surgery
Department of Surgery
Adjunct Clinical Assistant Professor
Department of Anatomy
University of Medicine and Dentistry of New Jersey
Robert Wood Johnson Medical School
New Brunswick, New Jersey

KENNETH S. KLEIN, M.D.
Associate Clinical Professor
Division of Orthopaedic Surgery
Department of Surgery
University of Medicine and Dentistry of New Jersey
Robert Wood Johnson Medical School
New Brunswick, New Jersey

RONG-ZENG LI, M.D.
Chief Illustrator

CHURCHILL LIVINGSTONE
New York, Edinburgh, London, Melbourne, Tokyo

Library of Congress Cataloging-in-Publication Data

Tria, Alfred J.
    An illustrated guide to the knee / Alfred J. Tria, Jr., Kenneth S.
Klein ; Rong-Zeng Li, chief illustrator.
        p. cm.
    Includes bibliographical references and index.
    ISBN 0-443-08794-6
    1. Knee—Atlases. 2. Knee—Diseases—Atlases. I. Klein, Kenneth
S. II. Title
    [DNLM: 1. Knee—atlases. 2. Knee Joint—atlases. WE 17 T819i]
    QM549.T75 1992
    617.5′82—dc20
    DNLM/DLC
    for Library of Congress   91-33942
                                                                  CIP

Distributed in the United Kingdom by Churchill Livingstone, Robert Stevenson House, 1–3
Baxter's Place, Leith Walk, Edinburgh EH1 3AF, and by associated companies, branches, and
representatives throughout the world.

Accurate indications, adverse reactions, and dosage schedules for drugs are provided in this
book, but it is possible that they may change. The reader is urged to review the package
information data of the manufacturers of the medications mentioned.

The Publishers have made every effort to trace the copyright holders for borrowed material. If
they have inadvertently overlooked any, they will be pleased to make the necessary arrange-
ments at the first opportunity.

Copy Editor: *Elizabeth Bowman-Schulman*
Production Designer: *Marci Jordan*
Production Supervisor: *Christina Hippeli*

Printed in the United States of America

First published in 1992   7 6 5 4 3 2 1

To Jeanne
A JT

To My Family
K SK

Preface

An Illustrated Guide to the Knee was begun almost four years ago when we realized that no text on the knee presented all the basic facts in one location. This book summarizes and reviews this primary information for the orthopaedic resident and the attending physician.

The text is intentionally brief to present the facts alone. The numerous illustrations by Rong-Zeng Li, an artist who is also a physician, and the tables present all the basic information in a concise, orderly format that is easy to use.

This book is not an attempt to establish a tome. All of the information it contains can be obtained by reviewing several other texts and sources and comparing materials. We have collated this information and organized it so that the reader may have the benefit of our time and, we hope, our experience.

The bibliographies at the end of each chapter are not meant to be definitive but do include most of the major publications, highlighting those that may be especially helpful.

We are grateful to Marsha E. Jessup and all the members of the Media Resources Department at Robert Wood Johnson Medical School for their tremendous support and patience.

Alfred J. Tria, Jr., M.D.
Kenneth S. Klein, M.D.

Contents

Anatomy

1

PHYLOGENY

Eryops, an amphibian that lived almost 320 million years ago, is believed to be the common ancestor of all reptiles, birds, and mammals. Its knee included a femorotibial and femorofibular articulation. The cruciate and collateral ligaments were present as were the menisci. With subsequent development, the femur rotated internally and the fibula receded distally away from the lateral femoral condyle (Fig. 1-1).

The osseous patella appeared last (approximately 65 million years ago).

EMBRYOLOGY

The basic outline of the knee is present in its entirety by the tenth week of gestation. The essential changes actually occur over an even shorter period (3 to 4 weeks).

Streeter's staging system outlined 23 horizons from the single cell to the end of the embryonic period (when the nutrient vessel penetrates the humerus) at approximately 7 weeks gestation (Fig. 1-2).

The limb bud appears in horizon 13 (28 days) as a mesodermal condensation. The ectoderm thickens and the mesodermal layer enlarges beneath this covering. At this point the leg bud is fin-like in appearance. By horizon 16 (33 days), the femur and the tibia and fibula begin to appear. A mesenchymal interzone then develops between the femur and tibia. At horizon 20 (41 days) the fibrous capsule appears. At horizon 22 (45 days) the patella is present, along with the cruciates, collaterals, and menisci.

By 9 to 10 weeks of age, the menisci separate from the articular surfaces and have developed attachments to the capsule (Fig. 1-3).

The epiphyses are visible by 36 weeks gestation. The times of appearance and closure of the epiphyses are summarized in Table 1-1. The female epiphyses appear sooner than their male counterparts and close off earlier. Only the distal femoral and proximal tibial plates are present at birth. The patella and proximal fibula appear next (approximately 3 to 4 years of age) followed by the tibial tuberosity at age 7 to 15 years. The patella can have many configurations; bi- and tri-partite are the most common variants. The secondary ossification center (bi-partite) is located superolaterally, is occasionally bilateral, and should not be confused with a fracture fragment. Marginal defects and duplications have also been recorded, but with much less frequency (Fig. 1-4).

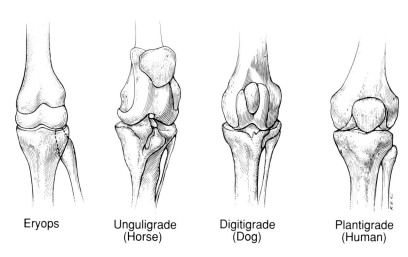

Eryops   Unguligrade (Horse)   Digitigrade (Dog)   Plantigrade (Human)

Fig. 1-1. Phylogenetic changes of the knee. (From Hosea TM, Bechler J, Tria AJ: Embryology of the knee. In Scott WN: Ligament and Extensor Mechanism Injuries of the Knee: Diagnosis and Treatment. CV Mosby, St. Louis, 1991, with permission.)

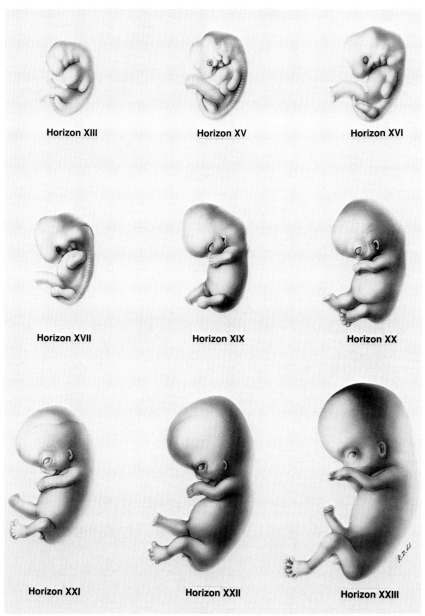

Horizon XIII   Horizon XV   Horizon XVI

Horizon XVII   Horizon XIX   Horizon XX

Horizon XXI   Horizon XXII   Horizon XXIII

Fig. 1-2. Embryologic development of the knee.

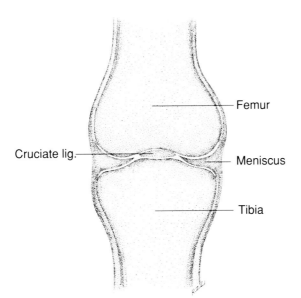

Fig. 1-3. Embryologic development of the menisci. (From Hosea TM, Bechler J, Tria AJ: Embryology of the knee. In Scott WN: Ligament and Extensor Mechanism Injuries of the Knee: Diagnosis and Treatment. CV Mosby, St. Louis, 1991, with permission.)

Patella fragmentations

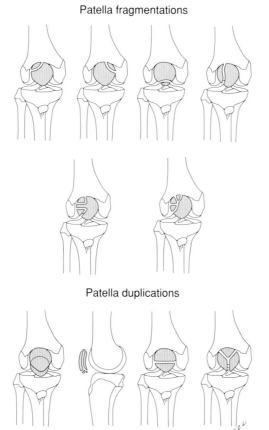

Patella duplications

Fig. 1-4. Anomalies of patellar development.

Table 1-1. Epiphyses of the Knee

	Appearance (yrs)		Closure (yrs)	
Epiphysis	Male	Female	Male	Female
Distal femur	(36th fetal week)		18/19	17
Proximal tibia	(40th fetal week)		18/19	16/17
Tibial tuberosity	7–15		19	
Proximal fibula	4	3	18/20	16/18
Patella	4/5	3		

(From Hosea TM, Bechler J, Tria AJ: Embryology of the knee. In Scott WN: Ligament and Extensor Mechanism Injuries of the Knee: Diagnosis and Treatment. CV Mosby, St. Louis, 1991, with permission.)

BONE STRUCTURE

The knee is a diarthrodial, tricompartmental joint consisting of a medial and lateral tibiofemoral and an anterior patellofemoral articulation (Fig. 1-5).

The medial femoral condyle is longer and larger than the lateral femoral condyle and has a larger circumference (Fig. 1-6). The width of the medial condyle at the level of the tibiofemoral articulation is slightly smaller than the lateral condyle. The two condyles diverge at an angle of 28 degrees from each other. (Fig. 1-7).

The lateral femoral condyle has a notch between the anterior one-third and the posterior two-thirds of the circumference. This notch separates the patellofemoral articulation from the tibiofemoral and clearly distinguishes the lateral condyle from the medial on a true lateral projection. The overall valgus of the knee is explained by the anteroposterior projection of the distal femur with the medial condyle extending distal to the lateral (Fig. 1-8).

The tibial plateau consists of two condyles (Fig. 1-9). The medial condyle is concave and wider from anterior to posterior than the lateral (Fig. 1-10). The

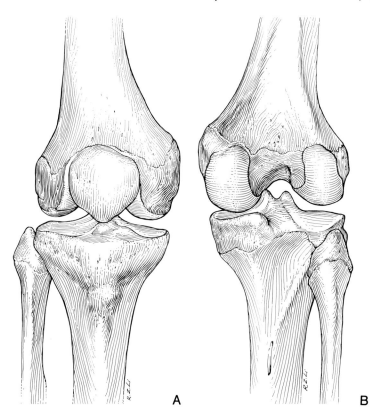

Fig. 1-5. (A) Anterior view of the right knee. (B) Posterior view of the right knee.

A   B

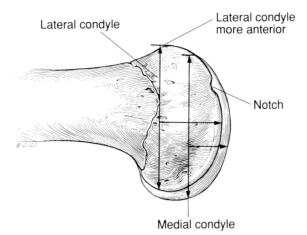

Fig. 1-6. Lateral view of the right knee.

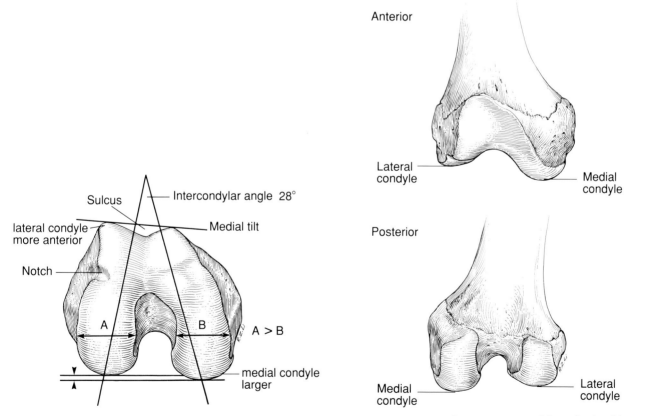

Fig. 1-7. Flexion view of the distal aspect of the right femur.

Fig. 1-8. Anterior and posterior view of the right distal femur.

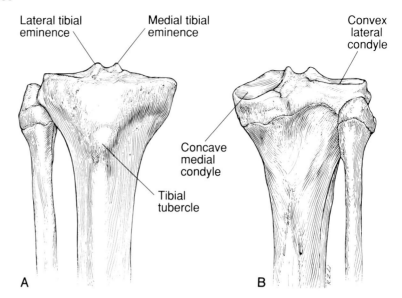

Fig. 1-9. (A) Anterior and (B) posterior view of the right proximal tibia.

A

B

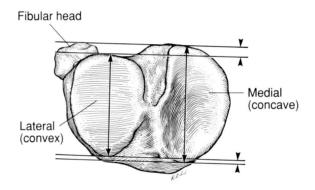

Fig. 1-10. Superior view of the right tibial plateau.

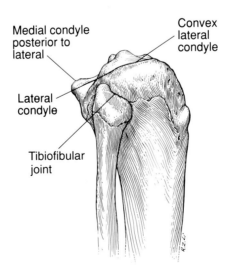

Fig. 1-11. Lateral view of the right proximal tibia.

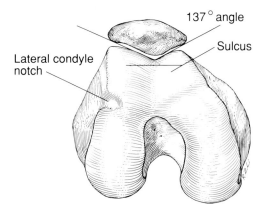

Fig. 1-12. Right patellofemoral articulation.

137° angle

Sulcus

Lateral condyle notch

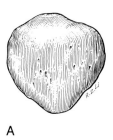

A

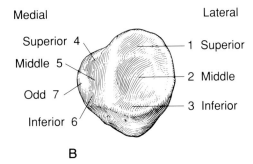

Medial

Superior 4

Middle 5

Odd 7

Inferior 6

Lateral

1 Superior

2 Middle

3 Inferior

B

Fig. 1-13. (A) Anterior and (B) posterior view of the patella.

lateral condyle is flat or convex. The medial condyle projects farther posterior and anterior than the lateral condyle on the true lateral view (Fig. 1-11). The tibial plateau surface has almost an oval appearance when seen from above. The tibial tubercle lies between the two condyles, usually in the midline, although sometimes it may be slightly externally rotated towards the lateral side.

The patellofemoral articulation includes the femoral sulcus and the posterior surface of the patella (Fig. 1-12). The distal margin of the sulcus can be identified by the notch on the lateral femoral condyle. Medially, the separation point is not as apparent. The sulcus angle is 137 degrees with a variation of 8 degrees. The entire sulcus is slightly internally rotated with respect to the femoral shaft. This is partially caused by the higher prominence of the lateral condyle.

The patellar surface can be divided into seven facets, three located medially, three laterally, and one above the medial facets (Fig. 1-13). The medial facets are usually smaller than the lateral and more convex than concave. The median ridge of the patella is located in the center of the femoral sulcus. It may be somewhat lateral to the midline but is almost never medial.

In earlier species the fibula articulates with the femur. With development, the fibula recedes distally and articulates only with the tibia. The proximal tibiofibular joint lies posterior to the metaphysis of the tibia and distal to the knee joint. Radiographic studies appear to show the joint as lateral to the tibia. This is not the case on anatomic dissection (see Fig. 1-11).

LIGAMENTS

There are four major ligamentous structures in the knee: the medial and the lateral collateral ligaments and the anterior and posterior cruciate ligaments. The collateral ligaments are extra-articular, whereas the two cruciate ligaments are intra-articular but extrasynovial.

The Collateral Ligaments

The medial collateral ligament originates from the medial femoral condyle at the adductor tubercle and descends distally and fans out as it inserts into the medial tibial metaphysis (Fig. 1-14). It appears sail-like and consists of two layers. The superficial layer follows the course outlined above. The deep layer originates from the femoral condyle slightly below the adductor tubercle and then proceeds distally to attach to the medial meniscus on its superior aspect. The ligament continues from the inferior aspect of the meniscus distally to blend into the superficial ligament along the medial tibial metaphysis.

The lateral collateral ligament originates from the lateral femoral condyle slightly posterior to its mid portion and descends to the fibula on its posterior aspect. The ligament is a thin structure almost strawlike in appearance (Fig. 1-15).

The Cruciate Ligaments

The cruciate ligaments are located in the central portion of the knee. They are covered by a synovial sheath that separates them from the intra-articular space and prevents synovial fluid from contacting the cruciate ligament surfaces (Fig. 1-16).

The anterior cruciate ligament consists of two bundles (Fig. 1-17). It originates from the lateral femoral condyle and proceeds distally to the anterior medial tibial plateau with a spiral rotation (Fig. 1-18). The anteromedial bundle is not as structurally significant as the posterolateral. The origin on the femoral condyle is oval and is almost horizontal when the knee is flexed to 90 degrees. This origin shifts to vertical when the knee is in full extension (Fig. 1-19). The tibial insertion is oval and slightly medial to midline on the anterior surface of the plateau (Fig. 1-20).

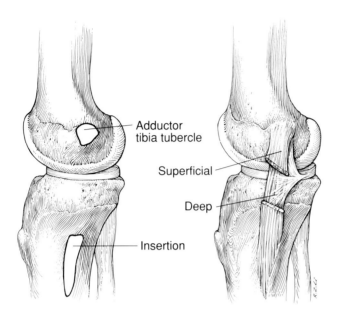

Fig. 1-14. The medial collateral ligament.

Adductor
tibia tubercle

Superficial

Deep

Insertion

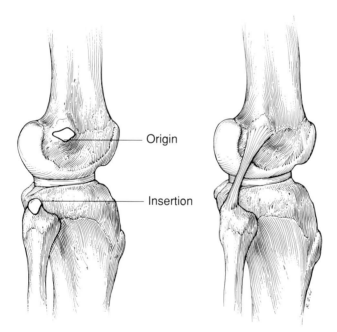

Origin

Insertion

Fig. 1-15. The lateral collateral ligament.

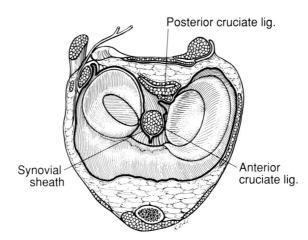

Fig. 1-16. The cruciate ligaments with their synovial relationship.

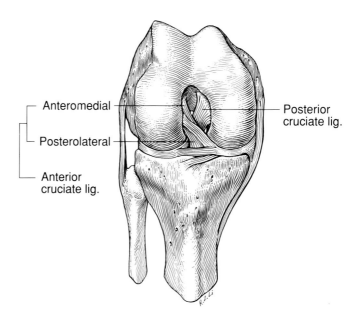

Fig. 1-17. Anterior view of the cruciates.

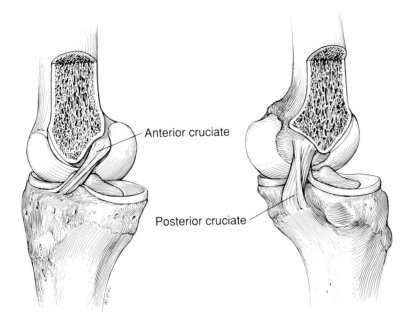

Fig. 1-18. Cutaway lateral view of the cruciates.

Anterior cruciate

Posterior cruciate

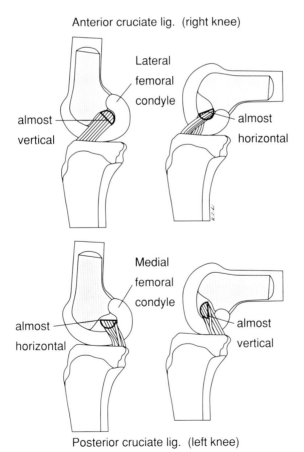

Anterior cruciate lig. (right knee)

Lateral femoral condyle

almost vertical

almost horizontal

Medial femoral condyle

almost horizontal

almost vertical

Posterior cruciate lig. (left knee)

Fig. 1-19. The relationship of the cruciate origins with flexion and extension of the knee.

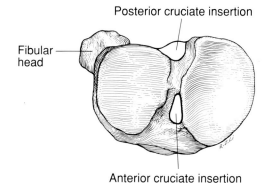

Posterior cruciate insertion

Fibular head

Anterior cruciate insertion

Fig. 1-20. Superior view of the insertions of the cruciates into the proximal tibial plateau.

The posterior cruciate ligament does not have any distinct bundles. It originates from the medial femoral condyle and inserts on the posterior surface of the tibial plateau in the midline (Fig. 1-17 and 1-18). Its origin on the medial femoral condyle is also oval and is 90 degrees offset from the anterior cruciate ligament origin. That is, the posterior cruciate ligament origin is horizontal with the knee in full extension and becomes vertical with 90 degrees of flexion of the knee (Fig. 1-19).

Other Ligaments

There are several lesser ligaments in the knee.

The patellofemoral ligaments extend from the medial and lateral facets and insert into the side of the medial and lateral femoral condyles. They are believed to help control tracking of the patella (Fig. 1-21).

Humphrey's ligament proceeds from the lateral meniscus across the anterior surface of the posterior cruciate ligament into the medial femoral condyle. Wrisberg's ligament lies posterior to the posterior cruciate and follows the same pattern from the lateral meniscus to the medial femoral condyle (Fig. 1-22).

The posterior aspect of the knee includes several ligaments that blend into the capsule. Beginning on the medial side, the posterior oblique ligament is a continuation of the insertion of the semi-membranosus into the tibia. It is a reflection superiorly from the medial aspect of the tibia into the posterior aspect of the medial collateral ligament. The oblique popliteal ligament extends across the posterior aspect of the knee from the inferomedial to the superolateral aspect (Fig. 1-23).

The lateral aspect of the knee consists of three layers, with the major contribution from the arcuate complex. The arcuate complex originates on the fibula and proceeds superomedially. The arcuate ligament extends across the posterior lateral aspect of the capsule and then blends into the midline. If a fabella is present (as either an osseous structure on the plain roentgenogram or as a cartilaginous anlage), then the fabellofibular ligament is the major ligament posterolaterally. If the fabella is absent, then the arcuate ligament is the major structure (see Fig. 1-23).

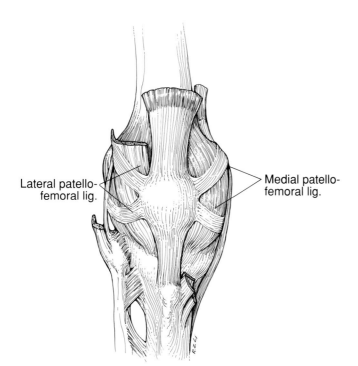

Fig. 1-21. The platellofemoral ligaments.

Lateral patello-femoral lig.

Medial patello-femoral lig.

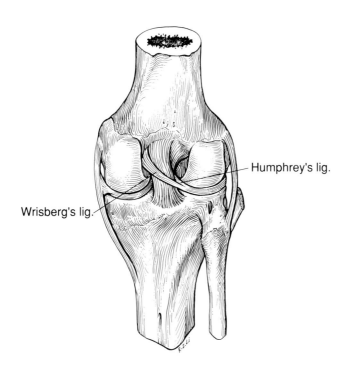

Fig. 1-22. The ligaments about the posterior cruciate.

Humphrey's lig.

Wrisberg's lig.

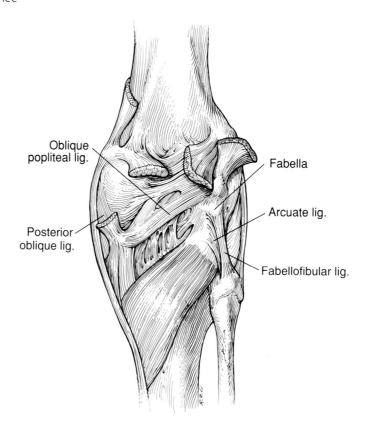

Oblique
popliteal lig.

Fabella

Arcuate lig.

Posterior
oblique lig.

Fabellofibular lig.

Fig. 1-23. The posterior ligaments of
the knee.

MENISCI

There are two menisci in the knee: medial and lateral. The embryologic
data indicate that the menisci develop during the fetal period and initially
appear to be C-shaped. There is no distinct data to indicate that the discoid
lateral meniscus is an embryologic aberrancy. The lateral meniscus is slightly
more circular than the medial.

The menisci are attached on the superior and inferior surfaces to the
capsule. The coronary ligaments are circular and proceed horizontally from
anterior to posterior around the periphery of the meniscus (Fig. 1-24). The
lateral meniscus has a defect in the attachment at the mid portion where the
popliteus tendon passes through from posteroinferior to anterosuperior to
attach to the lateral femoral condyle (Fig. 1-25). The tendon proceeds beneath the lateral collateral ligament and attaches just anterior to it on the
condyle. It is debatable whether the tendon has any attachment to the lateral
meniscus (Fig. 1-26). There are synovial pillars anterior and posterior to the
defect that enforce the capsular attachment to the lateral meniscus that may
protect the defect area from rupture. The lateral meniscus is subject to much
greater motion anterior to posterior than the medial meniscus, which has a
stronger attachment to the capsule and less excursion.

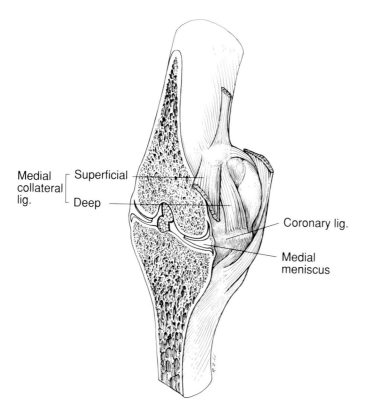

Medial collateral lig. ┌ Superficial
                       └ Deep

Coronary lig.

Medial meniscus

Fig. 1-24. Capsular and ligamentous attachments to the medial meniscus.

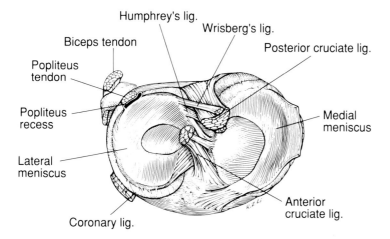

Humphrey's lig.

Wrisberg's lig.

Biceps tendon

Posterior cruciate lig.

Popliteus tendon

Popliteus recess

Medial meniscus

Lateral meniscus

Coronary lig.

Anterior cruciate lig.

Fig. 1-25. Superior view of the menisci.

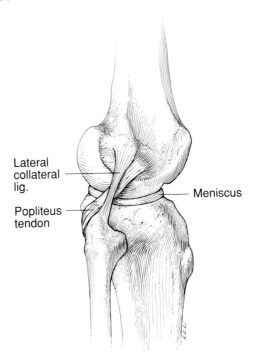

Fig. 1-26. Lateral view of the lateral meniscus.

Lateral collateral lig.

Popliteus tendon

Meniscus

PLICAE

Plicae are infoldings of the lining of the knee. They are not necessarily present in every knee and do not represent pathologic entities unless there is associated inflammation about the base. There are three synovial plicae. The supra patellar plica is circular in appearance and almost closes off the suprapatellar pouch when it is present (Fig. 1-27). The medial plica extends from the medial capsule at the level of the superior margin of the femoral condyle and traverses the medial joint space across to the patellar fat pad in the midline (Figs. 1-27 and 1-28). The ligamentum mucosum (the third plica) originates from the roof of the intercondylar notch and crosses to the patellar fat pad; this structure is important because it may be confused with the anterior cruciate ligament during the course of an arthroscopy (Figs. 1-27 and 1-29). The lateral recess of the knee also has a fold in it that mimics a plica but has not formerly been considered one (Figs. 1-27 and 1-28).

MUSCLES

The musculature of the knee can be divided into four major areas: the quadriceps (Fig. 1-30), the medial hamstrings (Fig. 1-31), the lateral hamstrings (Fig. 1-32), and the posterior gastroc-soleus complex (Fig. 1-33).

The quadriceps group forms the extensor mechanism of the knee. The intermedius muscle is wrapped about the anterior femoral shaft and is the deepest muscle of the group. The vastus medialis and lateralis are on either side of the intermedius and superior to it. The rectus femoris, the most superficial, inserts directly into the quadriceps tendon.

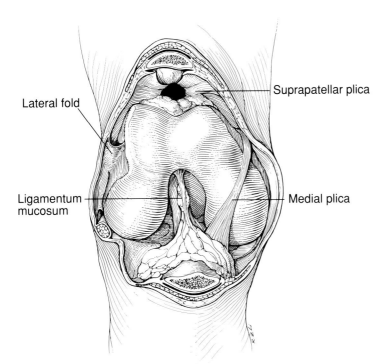

Fig. 1-27. Flexion view of the plicae.

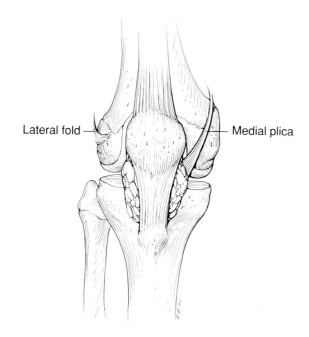

Fig. 1-28. Anterior view of the plicae.

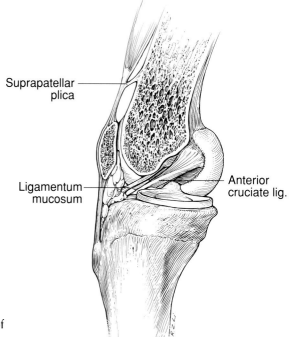

Suprapatellar
plica

Ligamentum
mucosum

Anterior
cruciate lig.

Fig. 1-29. Lateral cutaway view of
the plicae.

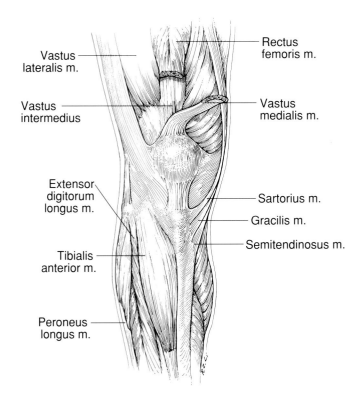

Vastus
lateralis m.

Rectus
femoris m.

Vastus
intermedius

Vastus
medialis m.

Extensor
digitorum
longus m.

Sartorius m.

Gracilis m.

Semitendinosus m.

Tibialis
anterior m.

Peroneus
longus m.

Fig. 1-30. The muscles of the anterior aspect of the knee.

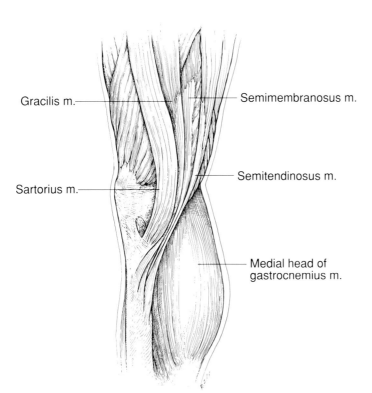

Gracilis m.

Semimembranosus m.

Semitendinosus m.

Sartorius m.

Medial head of
gastrocnemius m.

Fig. 1-31. The muscles of the medial
aspect of the knee.

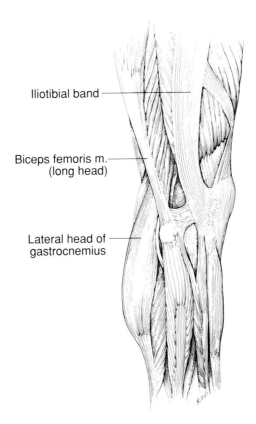

Iliotibial band

Biceps femoris m.
(long head)

Lateral head of
gastrocnemius

Fig. 1-32. The muscles of the lateral
aspect of the knee.

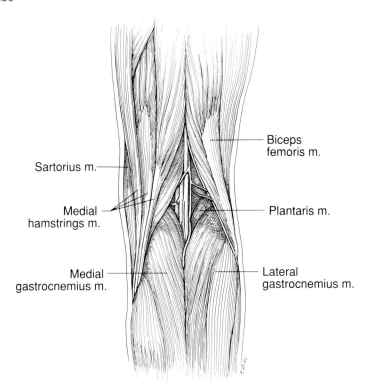

Sartorius m.

Medial
hamstrings m.

Medial
gastrocnemius m.

Biceps
femoris m.

Plantaris m.

Lateral
gastrocnemius m.

Fig. 1-33. The muscles of the posterior aspect of the knee.

The medial hamstrings include the gracilis, the semi-membranosus, and the semi-tendinosus. All have origins on the pelvis and insert on the medial side of the tibial metaphysis. They cause flexion and internal rotation.

The lateral hamstrings include the two heads of the biceps femoris (one from the pelvis and the other from the femoral shaft). This group leads to flexion and slight external rotation, but does not at all equal the force exerted by the medial group.

The remaining posterior muscle is the gastrocnemius soleus complex. The two heads of the gastrocnemius originate from the posterior aspect of the femoral condyles. They also contribute somewhat to flexion. The plantaris muscle originates from the posterior aspect of the lateral femoral condyle and inserts into the medial side of the calcaneus. The popliteus has its origin on the posterior tibial metaphysis and inserts into the lateral side of the lateral femoral condyle. Both of these smaller muscles may contribute slightly to flexion. The popliteus is also thought to cause rotation of the femoral condyle. Figures 1-34 and 1-35 illustrate the origin and insertion of the muscles.

VASCULATURE

The femoral artery divides into a deep and a superficial branch. The deep branch terminates in the upper thigh. The superficial branch continues distally into the adductor canal and spirals around the posterior aspect of the medial femoral condyle (Fig. 1-36).

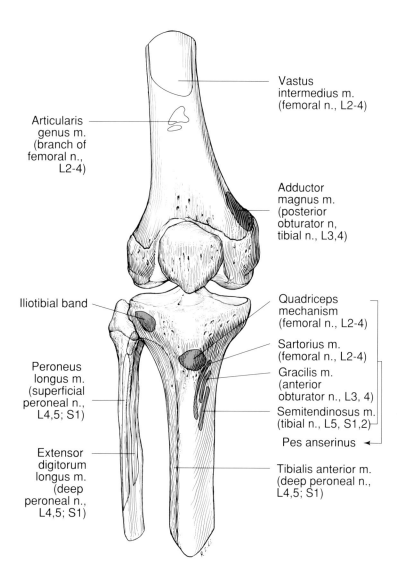

Vastus
intermedius m.
(femoral n., L2-4)

Articularis
genus m.
(branch of
femoral n.,
L2-4)

Adductor
magnus m.
(posterior
obturator n,
tibial n., L3,4)

Iliotibial band

Quadriceps
mechanism
(femoral n., L2-4)

Sartorius m.
(femoral n., L2-4)

Peroneus
longus m.
(superficial
peroneal n.,
L4,5; S1)

Gracilis m.
(anterior
obturator n., L3, 4)

Semitendinosus m.
(tibial n., L5, S1,2)

Pes anserinus ◄

Extensor
digitorum
longus m.
(deep
peroneal n.,
L4,5; S1)

Tibialis anterior m.
(deep peroneal n.,
L4,5; S1)

Fig. 1-34. Origin, insertion, and innervation of the anterior musculature.

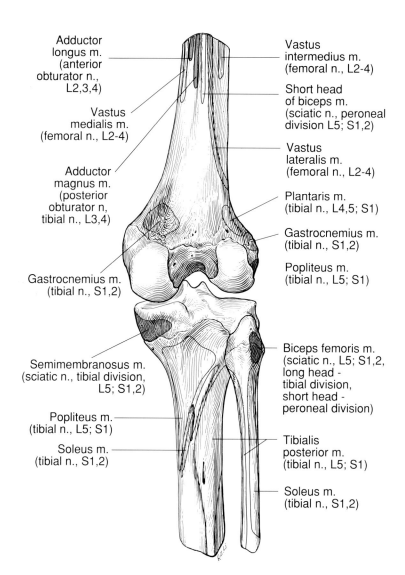

Adductor
longus m.
(anterior
obturator n.,
L2,3,4)

Vastus
medialis m.
(femoral n., L2-4)

Adductor
magnus m.
(posterior
obturator n,
tibial n., L3,4)

Gastrocnemius m.
(tibial n., S1,2)

Semimembranosus m.
(sciatic n., tibial division,
L5; S1,2)

Popliteus m.
(tibial n., L5; S1)

Soleus m.
(tibial n., S1,2)

Vastus
intermedius m.
(femoral n., L2-4)

Short head
of biceps m.
(sciatic n., peroneal
division L5; S1,2)

Vastus
lateralis m.
(femoral n., L2-4)

Plantaris m.
(tibial n., L4,5; S1)

Gastrocnemius m.
(tibial n., S1,2)

Popliteus m.
(tibial n., L5; S1)

Biceps femoris m.
(sciatic n., L5; S1,2,
long head -
tibial division,
short head -
peroneal division)

Tibialis
posterior m.
(tibial n., L5; S1)

Soleus m.
(tibial n., S1,2)

Fig. 1-35. Origin, insertion, and innervation of the posterior musculature.

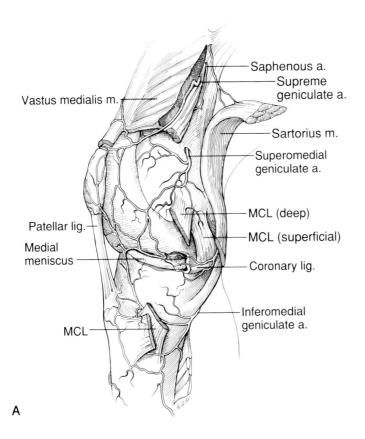

Saphenous a.

Supreme
geniculate a.

Vastus medialis m.

Sartorius m.

Superomedial
geniculate a.

MCL (deep)

Patellar lig.

MCL (superficial)

Medial
meniscus

Coronary lig.

Inferomedial
geniculate a.

MCL

A

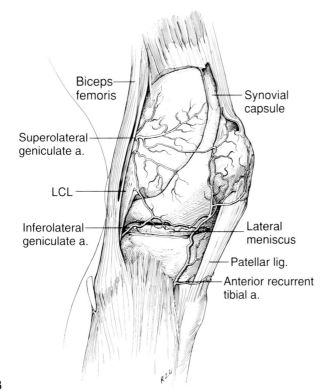

Biceps
femoris

Synovial
capsule

Superolateral
geniculate a.

LCL

Inferolateral
geniculate a.

Lateral
meniscus

Patellar lig.

Anterior recurrent
tibial a.

B

Fig. 1-36. (A) Medial vasculature of
the knee. (B) Lateral vasculature of
the knee.

There are seven major vessels that form the blood supply to the knee: the superolateral, superomedial, inferolateral, inferomedial, and middle geniculates take origin from the popliteal artery. The supreme geniculate originates from the superficial femoral artery and proceeds distally. The recurrent anterior tibial originates from the anterior tibial artery above the intraosseous membrane between the fibula and the tibia and proceeds proximally to the knee (Figs. 1-37 and 1-38). Of the five geniculates that take origin directly from the popliteal artery, the superolateral geniculate originates most superiorly, followed by the superomedial. The middle geniculate originates at the level of the joint line and supplies the anterior cruciate ligament. The inferolateral extends anteriorly along the lateral joint line, and the inferomedial is located 2 cm distal to the medial joint line along the metaphysis of the tibia.

Several of the vital structures within the knee joint have a tenuous blood supply that can easily be compromised. The patella is surrounded by a circular plexus of vessels. The majority of the blood supply is distally based, coming through the fat pad. Thus, a transverse fracture of the patella may cut off the proximal blood and lead to avascular necrosis.

The anterior cruciate supply comes from the femoral side through the overlying synovium from the middle geniculate. Injury to the synovial sheath can lead to loss of the ligament's integrity even without any significant mechanical injury to the ligament itself. The circulation to the posterior cruciate is entirely different, coming from the surrounding capsule and synovium, with a much broader base. Thus, vascular injury to the posterior cruciate is extremely rare.

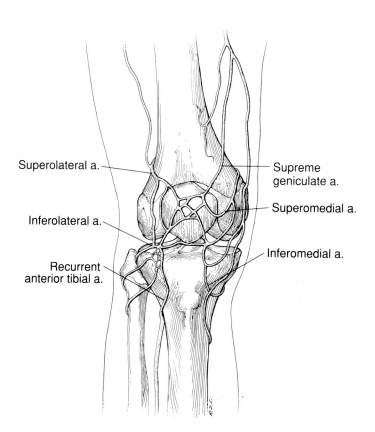

Fig. 1-37. Anterior vasculature of the knee.

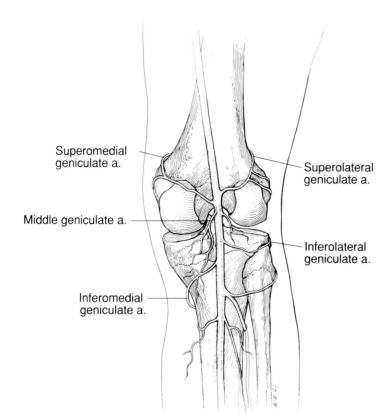

Superomedial geniculate a.

Superolateral geniculate a.

Middle geniculate a.

Inferolateral geniculate a.

Inferomedial geniculate a.

Fig. 1-38. Posterior vasculature of the knee.

The menisci are not nourished through the synovial fluid that surrounds them; rather, the vessels along the joint line derived from the inferolateral and inferomedial geniculates penetrate from the periphery to the inner edges. This explains why meniscal tears in the inner third of the body heal very poorly, if at all.

The blood supply to the distal femur and proximal tibia is less well understood and appears to depend upon the vasculature established for the original nourishment of the epiphyseal plates even after they are closed.

INNERVATION

The muscles about the knee are innervated by the nerve roots from L2 through S2.

The femoral nerve supplies the quadriceps group and the sartorius (Figs. 1-34 and 1-39). The sciatic nerve contains two major divisions, the tibial and peroneal. The tibial nerve supplies the large majority of the posterior and medial muscles about the knee. This group includes the long head of the biceps, semitendinosus, semimembranosus, plantaris, popliteus, gastrocnemius, and soleus. The single muscle innervated in the thigh by the peroneal nerve is the short head of the biceps femoris (Figs. 1-35 and 1-40).

The dermatomes of the lower extremities begin with L2 and extend to S2. They tend to spiral around the lower leg (Fig. 1-41).

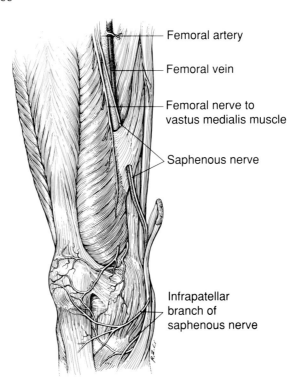

Femoral artery

Femoral vein

Femoral nerve to
vastus medialis muscle

Saphenous nerve

Infrapatellar
branch of
saphenous nerve

Fig. 1-39. Femoral nerve innervation anteriorly.

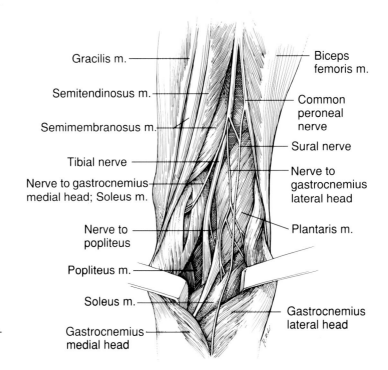

Gracilis m.

Semitendinosus m.

Semimembranosus m.

Tibial nerve

Nerve to gastrocnemius
medial head; Soleus m.

Nerve to
popliteus

Popliteus m.

Soleus m.

Gastrocnemius
medial head

Biceps
femoris m.

Common
peroneal
nerve

Sural nerve

Nerve to
gastrocnemius
lateral head

Plantaris m.

Gastrocnemius
lateral head

Fig. 1-40. Tibial and peroneal innervation posteriorly.

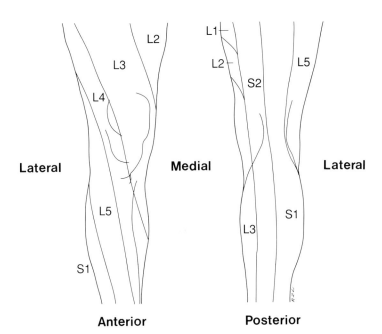

Fig. 1-41. The dermatomes of the lower leg.

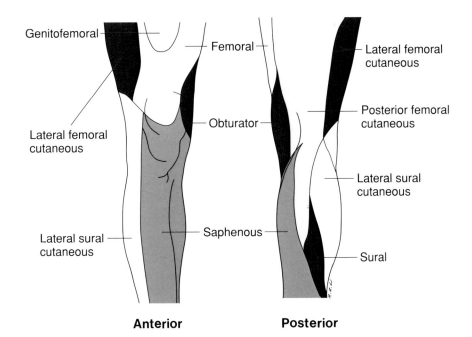

Fig. 1-42. Anterior and posterior cutaneous innervation.

The anterior cutaneous innervation begins medially from the obturator nerve and proceeds laterally to the femoral nerve, and then to the lateral femoral cutaneous. Just distal to this area, the saphenous nerve and the lateral sural cutaneous complete the anterior pattern.

The posterior cutaneous innervation is a continuation of the anteromedial and anterolateral coverage with the posterior femoral cutaneous covering the midline (Fig. 1-42).

SUGGESTED READINGS

Arnoczky SP, Rubin RM, Marshall JL: Microvasculature of the cruciate ligaments and its response to injury. An experimental study in dogs. J Bone Joint Surg [Am] 1979 Dec;61(8):1221 – 9

**Arnoczky SP: Anatomy of the anterior cruciate ligament. Clin Orthop 1983 Jan-Feb;(172):19 – 25

Barrett GR, Tomasin JD: Bilateral congenital absence of the anterior cruciate ligament. Orthopedics 1988 Mar;11(3):431 – 4

*Carlson DH, O'Connor J: Congenital dislocation of the knee. Am J Roentgenol 1976 Sep;127(3):465 – 8

*Dye SF, Cannon WD Jr: Anatomy and biomechanics of the anterior cruciate ligament. Clin Sports Med 1988 Oct;7(4):715 – 25

Ellison AE, Berg EE: Embryology, anatomy, and function of the anterior cruciate ligament. Orthop Clin North Am 1985 Jan;16(1):3 – 14

Ferrone JD Jr: Congenital lateral dislocation of the patella. J Bone Joint Surg [Br] 1968 May;50(2):285 – 9

Fuss FK: Anatomy of the cruciate ligaments and their function in extension and flexion of the human knee joint. Am J Anat 1989 Feb;184(2):165 – 76

Girgis FG, Marshall JL, Monajem A: The cruciate ligaments of the knee joint. Anatomical, functional and experimental analysis. Clin Orthop 1975 Jan-Feb;(106):216 – 31

Gronblad M, Korkala O, Liesi P, Karaharju E: Innervation of synovial membrane and meniscus. Acta Orthop Scand 1985 Dec;56(6):484 – 6

Grood ES, Hefzy MS, Lindenfield TN: Factors affecting the region of most isometric femoral attachments. Part I: The posterior cruciate ligament. Am J Sports Med 1989 Mar-Apr;17(2):197 – 207

Hefzy MS, Grood ES, Noyes FR: Factors affecting the region of most isometric femoral attachments. Part II: The anterior cruciate ligament. Am J Sports Med 1989 Mar-Apr;17(2):208 – 16

Katz MP, Grogono BJ, Soper KC: The etiology and treatment of congenital dislocation of the knee. J Bone Joint Surg [Br] 1967 Feb;49(1):112 – 20

Johansson E, Aparisi T: Congenital absence of the cruciate ligaments: a case report and review of the literature. Clin Orthop 1982 Jan-Feb;(162):108 – 11

*Kennedy JC, Alexander IJ, Hayes KC: Nerve supply of the human knee and its functional importance. Am J Sports Med 1982 Nov-Dec;10(6):329 – 35

Kennedy JC, Grainger RW: The posterior cruciate ligament. J Trauma 1967 May;7(3):367 – 77

**Kennedy JC, Weinberg HW, Wilson AS: The anatomy and function of the anterior cruciate ligament. As determined by clinical and morphological studies. J Bone Joint Surg [Am] 1974 Mar;56(2):223 – 35

Mayfield GW: Popliteus tendon tenosynovitis. Am J Sports Med 1977 Jan-Feb;5(1):31 – 6

Odensten M, Gillquist J: Functional anatomy of the anterior cruciate ligament and a rationale for reconstruction. J Bone Joint Surg [Am] 1985 Feb;67(2):257 – 62

Ogden JA: The anatomy and function of the proximal tibiofibular joint. Clin Orthop 1974 Jun;101(01):186 – 91

** Source reference
* Reference of major interest

Rauschning W: Popliteal cysts and their relation to the gastrocnemio-semimembran-
osus bursa. Studies on the surgical and functional anatomy. Acta Orthop Scand
Suppl 1979;179:1–43

Reider B, Marshall JL, Warren RF: Persistant vertical septum in the human knee joint. J
Bone Joint Surg [Am] 1981 Sep;63A(7):1185–7

*Reider B, Marshall JL, Koslin B et al: The anterior aspect of the knee joint. J Bone Joint
Surg [Am] 1981 Mar;63A(3):351–6

Schutte MJ, Dabezies EJ, Zimny ML, Happel NV: Neural anatomy of the human
anterior cruciate ligament. J Bone Joint Surg [Am] 1987 Feb;69(2):243–7

*Seebacher JR, Inglis AE, Marshall JL, Warren RF: The structure of the posterolateral
aspect of the knee. J Bone Joint Surg [Am] 1982 Apr;64(4):536–41

Thomas NP, Jackson AM, Aichroth PM: Congenital absence of the anterior cruciate
ligament. A common component of knee dysplasia. J Bone Joint Surg [Br] 1985
Aug;67(4):572–5

Tria AJ Jr, Johnson CD, Zawadsky JP: The popliteus tendon. J Bone Joint Surg [Am]
1989 Jun;71(5):714–6

Van Dommelen BA, Fowler PJ: Anatomy of the posterior cruciate ligament. A review.
Am J Sports Med 1989 Jan-Feb;17(1):24–9

*Warren LF, Marshall JL: The supporting structures and layers on the medial side of the
knee: an anatomical analysis. J Bone Joint Surg [Am] 1979 Jan;61(1):56–62

Biomechanics **2**

MECHANICAL ANATOMY

Motion of the knee occurs in three planes. The nature of the motion is best understood by referring to the underlying bony anatomy discussed in Chapter 1.

The femoral condyles are asymmetric. They have spiral centers of rotation; the medial femoral condyle center is posterior and inferior to the center of the lateral femoral condyle rotation. The medial condyle is larger than the lateral; however, the coronal width of the lateral condyle is larger than the medial. The patellofemoral articulation is tilted medially because the anterior aspect of the lateral condyle is higher than that of the medial. The circumference of the medial condyle is more circular and uniform than the lateral condyle, which tends to be slightly flattened secondary to the notch (Fig. 2-1).

The medial and lateral condyles of the tibia are also asymmetric with a concave medial and a convex lateral surface. The circumference is oval with the medial side larger and projecting equally anterior and posterior to the lateral side. The medial tibial eminence is slightly anterior to the lateral, and they both lend some constraint to the medial and lateral femoral condyles (Figs. 2-2 – 2-4).

The fibular head articulates with the proximal posterolateral tibial metaphysis and does not enter into the mechanics of the joint.

The articular surface of the patella occupies the proximal two-thirds of the total body of the patella (Fig. 2-5).

KINEMATICS

As knee motion proceeds from full extension to flexion, the contact point of the femur on the tibia moves posteriorly. This motion is a combination of point to point and some slide (Figs. 2-6 and 2-7). Because of the larger, longer medial femoral condyle and medial tibial plateau surfaces (versus the lateral compartment), the distance traversed on the medial side is greater than that traversed on the lateral aspect; therefore, the tibia internally rotates on the femur as flexion occurs. The reverse occurs as the knee progresses from flexion into extension and explains the *screw-home* of the tibia on the femur. At terminal extension the tibia externally rotates and locks into position beneath the femur (Fig. 2-8).

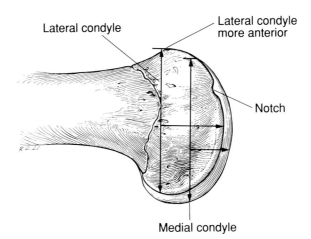

Fig. 2-1. Lateral view of the right distal femur.

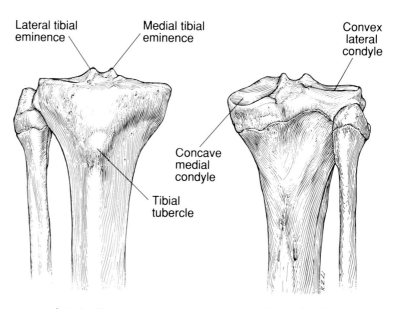

Fig. 2-2. Anterior and posterior view of the right proximal tibia.

Anterior View   Posterior view

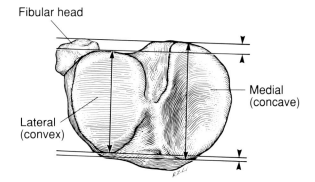

Fig. 2-3. Superior view of the right tibial plateau.

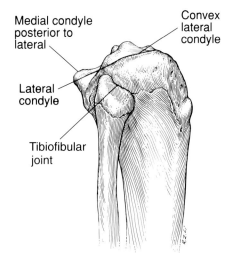

Fig. 2-4. Lateral view of the right proximal tibia.

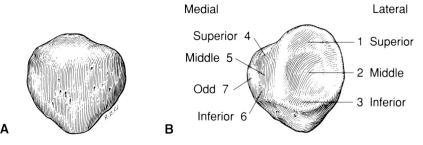

Fig. 2-5. (A) Anterior view of the patella and (B) posterior view showing the seven facets of the articular surface.

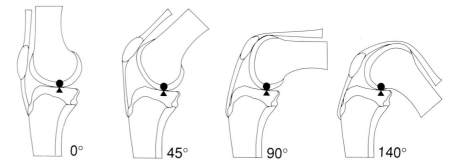

Fig. 2-6. Posterior shift of the tibio-femoral contact point with flexion of the knee.

FLEXION

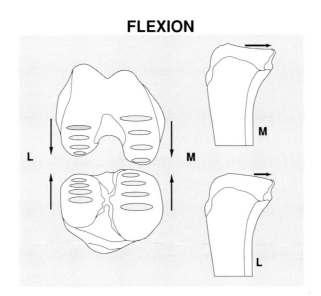

Fig. 2-7. The surface contact between the femur and the tibia moves posteriorly with flexion. There is a larger distance traversed on the medial side than on the lateral.

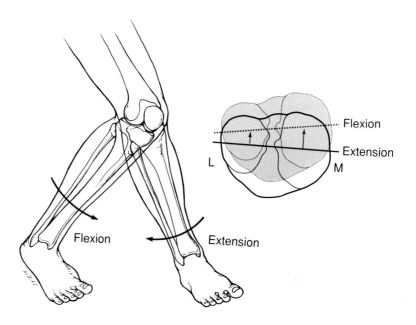

Fig. 2-8. The tibia externally rotates with extension and internally rotates with flexion of the knee.

Some believe that the musculature also contributes to the screw home and implicate the popliteus muscle, the hamstrings, and iliotibial band insertion into Gerdy's tubercle. As the knee enters full extension, the popliteus and the iliotibial band encourage external rotation. As the knee flexes, the medial hamstrings rotate the tibia internally.

The ligaments do effect the rotation but to a lesser extent than the bony architecture. The medial collateral origin on the femoral condyle is in the midline from anterior to posterior, whereas the lateral collateral is slightly posterior to the midline. This cooperates with the asymmetric motion and encourages the contact to move posterior (Figs. 2-9 and 2-10). The spiral nature of the cruciates allows them to unroll with flexion and extension to permit the internal and external rotation of the tibia.

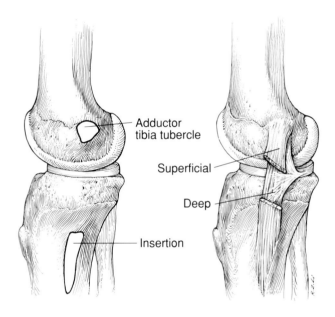

Fig. 2-9. The medial collateral ligament lies in the midline from anterior to posterior on both the femur and the tibia.

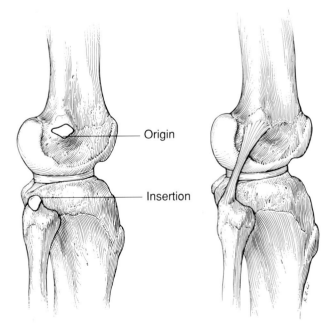

Fig. 2-10. The lateral collateral ligament originates from the midportion of the femur and proceeds posteriorly to the fibular head.

The Patellofemoral Joint

The patella does not articulate with the sulcus of the femur when the knee is in full extension. Contact begins at about 30 degrees of flexion with the distal central ridge articulating with the surface of the sulcus of the femur. Because of the oblique pull of the quadriceps mechanism, and the higher lateral femoral sulcus area, the patella begins flexion slightly on the lateral side of the sulcus (tilted). This lateral tilt position gradually corrects itself as further flexion occurs. The medial and lateral facets of the patella begin to contact the opposing femoral surfaces at about 45 degrees of flexion. This contact starts on the distal portions of the patella and proceeds proximally on the patellar facets as flexion continues. At extreme flexion, the patella is locked in the midline and the odd facet can contact the medial femoral condyle. The contact zones on the sulcus of the femur progress distally with flexion and spread to the medial and lateral condylar areas (Fig. 2-11).

Joint Reaction Forces

The forces across the femorotibial joint can exceed four to six times the total body weight. The menisci participate in relieving some of the stress on the articular surfaces by increasing the contact area (stress is defined as force divided by area). The collagen fibers, arranged radially and circumferentially, permit the meniscus to "expand" under compressive forces and thus increase the effective area of contact (Fig. 2-12). The two fibrocartilages can also slide anteroposteriorly to permit the roll back into flexion and still maintain similar surface contact. Finally, the fibrocartilaginous material has some visco-elasticity to help absorb energy over time.

The patella acts as a fulcrum for the quadriceps mechanism. It increases the distance of the lever arm from the center of rotation of the knee and thus improves the mechanical advantage of the quadriceps (Fig. 2-13). Because of the small area of the patellar facets and the lack of menisci to increase the area of contact, the surface is subject to slightly higher forces (up to eight times body weight) than the femorotibial surfaces.

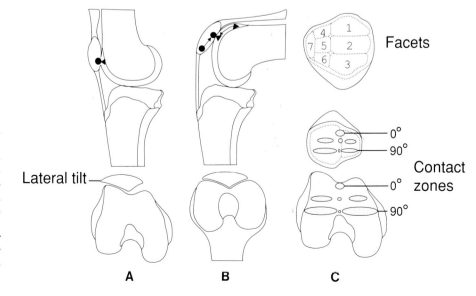

Fig. 2-11. (A) In extension the patella sits slightly lateral in the femoral sulcus, and the distal patellar articular surface is in contact with the femur. (B) As flexion progresses, the patella reduces into the sulcus of the femur, and the contact zone on the patella shifts proximally. (C) As the knee flexes, the patellar surface contact spreads medially and laterally onto the femoral surfaces.

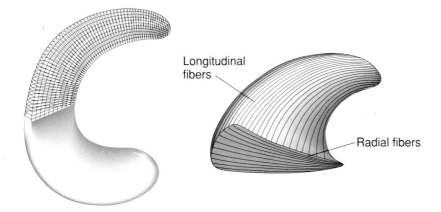

Fig. 2-12. The collagen fibers of the meniscus are arranged in both a radial and circumferential fashion.

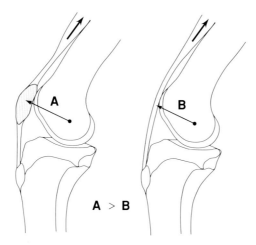

Fig. 2-13. The patella increases the moment arm of the quadriceps mechanism, thus improving its mechanical advantage.

Viscosity and Fluid Mechanics

The total synovial fluid in the joint is less than one cubic centimeter. It does, however, decrease frictional forces through the range of motion and helps to increase the total area of contact in the femorotibial joint (once again decreasing the stress). These two functions are accomplished because of the fluid's frequency-dependent visco-elasticity. As the sheer frequency increases, the synovial fluid changes from a viscous liquid to an elastic solid.

SUGGESTED READINGS

Cabaud HE: Biomechanics of the anterior cruciate ligament. Clin Orthop 1983 Jan-Feb;(172):26 – 31

**Frankel VH: Biomechanics of the knee. Orthop Clin North Am 1971 Mar;2(1):175 – 90

** Source reference
* Reference of major interest

Hsu RW, Himeno S, Coventry MB, Chảo EY: Normal axial alignment of the lower extremity and load-bearing distribution at the knee. Clin Orthop 1990 Jun;(255):215–27

*Hungerford DS, Barry M: Biomechanics of the patellofemoral joint. Clin Orthop 1979 Oct;(144):9–15

Kaufer H: Patellar biomechanics. Clin Orthop 1979 Oct;(144):51–4

Matthews LS, Sonstegard DA, Henke JA: Load bearing characteristics of the patello-femoral joint. Acta Orthop Scand 1977;48(5):511–6

Nissan M: Review of some basic assumptions in knee biomechanics. J Biomech 1980;13(4):375–81

**Noyes FR, Grood ES: The strength of the anterior cruciate ligament in humans and Rhesus monkeys. J Bone Joint Surg [Am] 1976 Dec;58(8):1074–82

Radin EL: Biomechanics of the knee joint. Its implications in the design of replacements. Orthop Clin North Am 1973 Apr;4(2):539–46

Reilly DT, Martens M: Experimental analysis of the quadriceps muscle force and patello-femoral joint reaction force for various activities. Acta Orthop Scand 1972;43(2):126–37

Reuben JD, Rovick JS, Schrager RJ et al: Three-dimensional dynamic motion analysis of the anterior cruciate ligament deficient knee joint. Am J Sports Med 1989 Jul-Aug;17(4):463–71

Smidt GL: Biomechanical analysis of knee flexion and extension. J Biomech 1973;6:79–82

Shrive NG, O'Connor JJ, Goodfellow JW: Load-bearing in the knee joint. Clin Orthop 1978 Mar-Apr;(131):279–87

Welsh RP: Knee joint structure and function. Clin Orthop 1980 Mar-Apr;(147):7–14

Physical Examination 3

HISTORY

A thorough orthopaedic evaluation should be preceded by a complete history. This information often suggests the areas of involvement in the knee or in the case of trauma may describe the mechanism of injury. The data may often lead one to suspect the anatomy of the physical examination before it is even initiated.

OBSERVATION AND INSPECTION

The physical examination of the knee should begin with evaluation of the gait pattern and observation of the standing attitude of the entire lower limb and then that of the knee. Any component of antalgia readily indicates the involved side. The varus or valgus alignment should be noted along with any medial or lateral thrust in the stance phase of gait (Fig. 3-1). The clinical alignment of the lower leg (anatomic axis) measures the femorotibial angle (Fig. 3-2) and differs from the mechanical axis of the limb (Fig. 3-3) as measured from the femoral head through the knee into the ankle on a standing roentgenogram.

The patellar alignment and the rotation of the forefoot are influenced by femoral neck anteversion (Fig. 3-4), tibial torsion (Fig. 3-5), and the presence or absence of metatarsus adductus. The Q angle is a measure of the overall rotational alignment effect upon the knee (Fig. 3-6). As the knee progresses from full extension to flexion, the Q angle decreases with the internal rotation of the tibia on the femur (Fig. 3-7).

A clinical effusion may be visually apparent. The active range of motion can be noted, with any limitations to full extension or flexion recorded for evaluation later in the examination (Fig. 3-8). Inability to fully extend may represent a lag, a locked knee, or a flexion contracture. Inability to fully flex may be due to an effusion, pain, or an extension contracture.

Quadriceps atrophy is sometimes visually apparent.

Figures 3-1, 3-8, and 3-12 through 3-25 are reproduced from Hosea TM, Tria AJ: Physical examination of the knee: clinical. In Scott WN: Ligament and Extensor Mechanism Injuries of the Knee: Diagnosis and Treatment. CV Mosby, St. Louis, 1991, with permission.

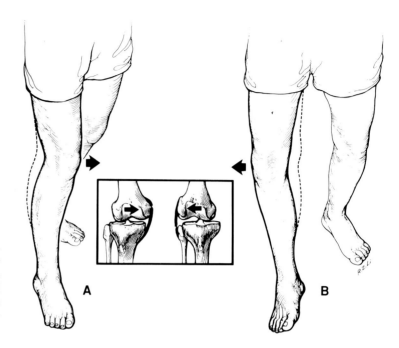

Fig. 3-1. (A) A medial thrust of the femur indicates shift of the femur medially on the tibia through the stance phase of gait in the coronal plane. (B) A lateral thrust indicates lateral shift of the femur in the coronal plane.

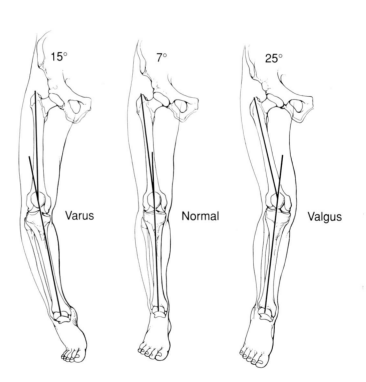

15°   7°   25°

Varus   Normal   Valgus

Fig. 3-2. The anatomic axis is measured by drawing lines parallel to the long axis of the femur and the tibia and measuring the intercepting angle.

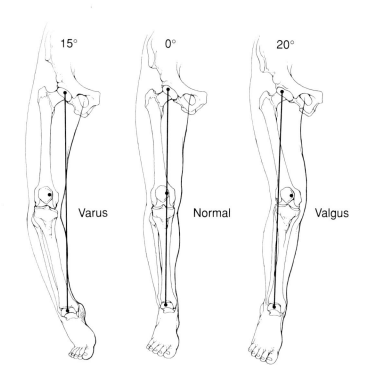

Fig. 3-3. The mechanical axis of the leg is measured in the standing position with an imaginary plumbline dropped from the femoral head to the ground. This angular measurement gives the best functional evaluation of the lower extremity alignment.

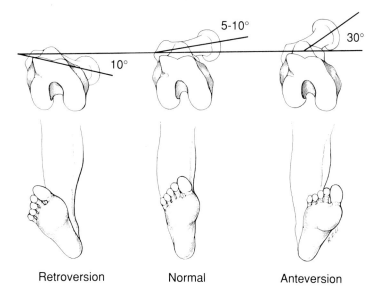

Fig. 3-4. Femoral neck anteversion measures the angle between the neck of the femur and the shaft of the bone. It leads to positioning of the foot as illustrated.

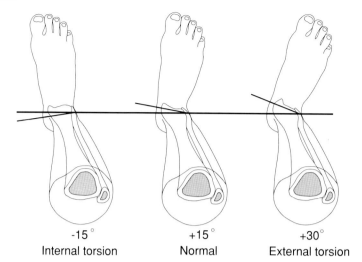

Fig. 3-5. Tibial torsion relates the rotation of the malleoli of the ankle to the tibial tubercle. Internal torsion rotates the malleoli internally along with the foot. External torsion rotates the malleoli externally along with the foot.

-15°
Internal torsion

+15°
Normal

+30°
External torsion

PALPATION

All of the bony landmarks should be palpated and identified. The Q angle is the angle between the line from the anterior superior iliac spine to the middle of the patella and the line from the middle of the patella to the middle of tibial tubercle. Gerdy's tubercle, the fibular head, the adductor tubercle of the femur, the patellar facets, and the femorotibial joint lines should all be identified (Fig. 3-7).

Effusions can be graded in size by compressing the supra patellar pouch and then noting any fluid (grade 1); slight lift-off of the patella (grade 2); a ballottable patella (grade 3); or a tense effusion with no ability to even compress the patella against the femoral sulcus (grade 4) (Fig. 3-9).

The muscle atrophy noted on observation can now be quantitated. The circumference of the thigh can be measured at a set number of centimeters above the patella with the knee in full extension. The calf can be measured by its greatest circumference in the lower leg.

Patellofemoral Joint

The examination includes both a static and a dynamic evaluation. The tracking of the patella from full extension into flexion should be visually recorded. In full extension the patella begins with contact of the median ridge and the lateral facet with the lateral side of the sulcus. The patella moves more centrally and the facets increase their contact with the femoral condyles as flexion increases (Fig. 3-10).

Because the patellar facets do not begin to contact the femoral sulcus until the knee is flexed 30 degrees, the medial and lateral patellofemoral articulation should be palpated in this degree of flexion. One should evaluate tenderness of each facet, apprehension with either medial or lateral compression, and any evidence of crepitation.

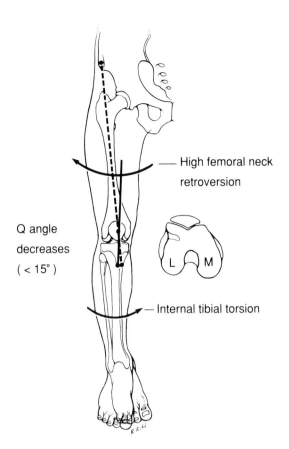

A

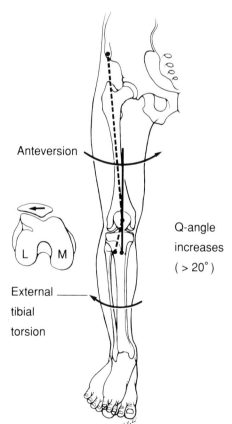

B

Fig. 3-6. (A) High femoral neck retroversion rotates the distal femur externally. In combination with internal tibial torsion, the Q angle is decreased. The patellar tracking is improved and patellofemoral sulcus alignment is normal. (B) High femoral neck anteversion rotates the distal femur internally. In combination with external tibial torsion, the Q angle is increased. Patellar tracking is compromised and the patella tends to track laterally.

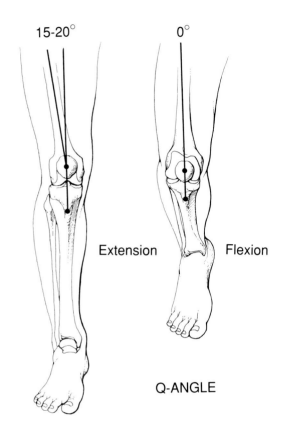

15-20°   0°

Extension   Flexion

Q-ANGLE

Fig. 3-7. Flexion of the knee decreases the Q angle because of the internal tibial rotation.

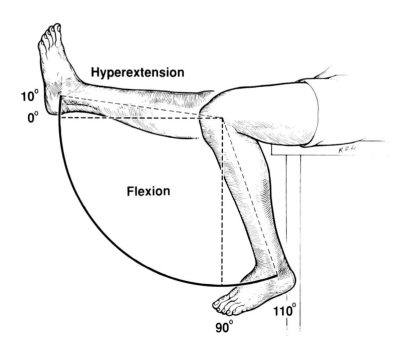

Hyperextension

10°

0°

Flexion

90°   110°

Fig. 3-8. Full extension of the knee is the zero or neutral point.

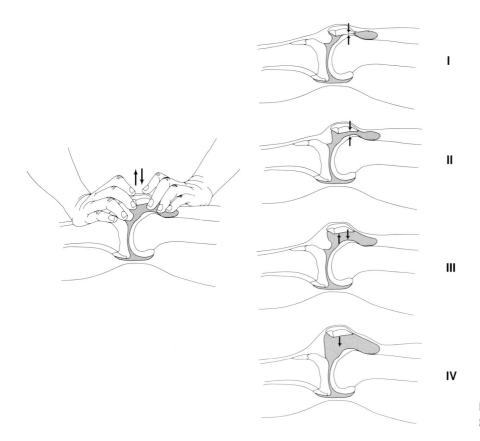

Fig. 3-9. Effusions of the knee are graded from one to four.

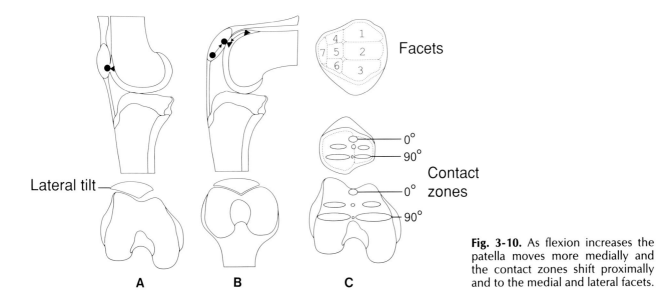

Fig. 3-10. As flexion increases the patella moves more medially and the contact zones shift proximally and to the medial and lateral facets.

Femorotibial Joint

The tibiofemoral examination should note the presence of any cystic mass (ganglion) along the joint line, localized tenderness, crepitation, snapping, or clicking.

Meniscal tears occur as a result of trauma to or degeneration of the fibro-cartilage. There may be symptoms of pain along the joint line when the knee is subjected to rotation. The physical examination of the knee with a torn meniscus elicits findings of joint line tenderness, palpable clicks, or snaps. One should initially note the range of motion as discussed above since a block to full extension may belie a torn meniscus with displacement and mechanical interference with tibiofemoral rotation.

The tests for meniscal tears can be divided into two groups: those that depend upon palpation to elicit tenderness or clicks, and those that depend upon symptoms of joint line pain with rotation (Table 3-1).

The primary palpation tests are Bragard's, McMurray's, and Steinmann's second sign.

Bragard's palpates the joint line and demonstrates that external tibial rotation and knee extension increases the tenderness of the torn medial meniscus. This test brings the meniscus anterior and closer to the examining finger. Internal rotation and flexion shows less tenderness. If the articular surfaces were the cause of these findings, then, there would be no difference between the two positions.

The McMurray test demonstrates a palpable click on the joint line. Medially, this is demonstrated with external tibial rotation and the range from flexion to extension. Laterally, it is demonstrated with the tibia in internal rotation and the range from flexion to extension. If the click is palpated in the initial degrees from full flexion, some examiners believe that the tear is more posterior. If the click is palpated later as the knee is brought into more extension, the tear is felt to be more anterior.

Steinmann's second test demonstrates joint line tenderness that moves posteriorly with knee flexion and anteriorly with knee extension. This is consistent with a meniscal tear that moves with the range of motion of the knee and not with joint line pathology that should remain stationary throughout the range of motion (Fig. 3-11A).

The remainder of the tests depend upon pain with rotation. The Apley grind forces the femorotibial surfaces together to elicit pain. This is believed to confirm a meniscal tear. The Apley, performed with the knee surfaces distracted, is believed to demonstrate lesions of the capsule or ligaments without meniscal involvement.

Table 3-1. Meniscal Tests
Palpation
Bragard's
McMurray
Steinmann's 2nd
Rotation
Apley
Apley Grind
Bohler's
Duck Walking
Helfet's
Merke's
Payr's
Steinmann's 1st

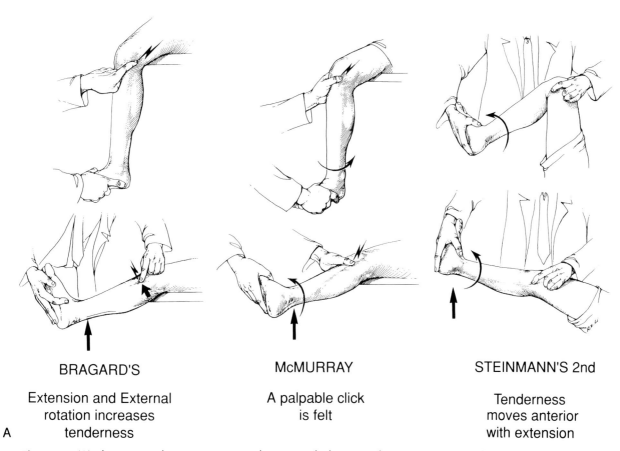

BRAGARD'S

Extension and External
rotation increases
tenderness

McMURRAY

A palpable click
is felt

STEINMANN'S 2nd

Tenderness
moves anterior
with extension

A

Fig. 3-11. (A) The meniscal tests requiring palpation include Bragard's, McMurray's, and Steinmann's second test. *(Fig. 3-11 continues)*

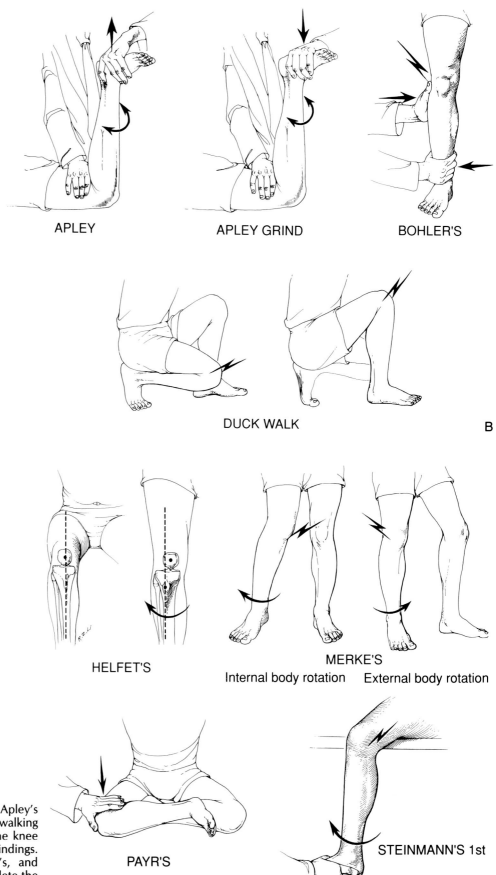

APLEY

APLEY GRIND

BOHLER'S

DUCK WALK

B

HELFET'S

MERKE'S

Internal body rotation

External body rotation

PAYR'S

STEINMANN'S 1st

Fig. 3-11 (Continued). (B) Apley's tests, Bohler's test, and duck walking depend upon rotation of the knee joint to elicit the meniscal findings. (C) Helfet's, Merke's, Payr's, and Steinmann's first tests complete the rotary tests for the meniscus.

C

Bohler's test is performed with varus stress to demonstrate a medial tear with compression (a lateral tear is diagnosed with valgus stress). Duck walking increases the compressive forces on the posterior horns of the torn menisci, thus causing pain.

Helfet's test is most helpful when the knee is locked. Because there is a mechanical block to the normal motion, the tibial tubercle cannot externally rotate with extension and the Q angle cannot increase to normal with extension of the knee.

Merke's test is merely the first Steinmann test with the patient in the weight-bearing position. Pain with internal rotation of the body produces external rotation of the tibia and medial joint line pain when the medial meniscus is torn. The opposite occurs when the lateral meniscus is torn.

Payr's test is performed with the patient in the "Turkish sitting position" and with downward force applied to the knee, resulting in medial pain with a torn medial meniscus.

Steinmann's first sign is a test done with the knee flexed to 90 degrees and sudden external rotation of the tibia for the medial meniscus. This results in pain along the medial joint line. Internal tibial rotation is utilized for the lateral meniscal tears (Fig. 3-11B and C).

STRESS EXAMINATION

The stress examination evaluates the four major ligaments along with the associated posteromedial and posterolateral capsular structures. The valgus stress examination in full extension includes the medial collateral ligament and the associated posteromedial capsule. In 30 degrees of flexion the same stress isolates the collateral by relaxing the capsule (Fig. 3-12). Thus, full extension evaluates the ligament and capsule; flexion evaluates the ligament alone. The varus examination should also include extension and flexion stress to evaluate the lateral collateral ligament and posterolateral capsule status (Fig. 3-13).

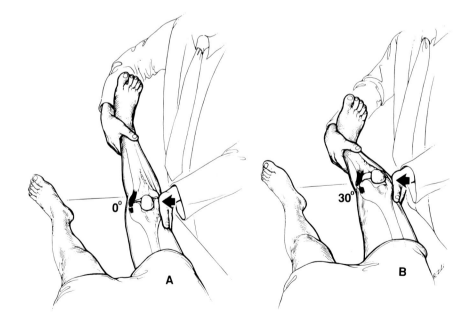

Fig. 3-12. The valgus stress in extension tests the medial collateral ligament and the posteromedial capsule. Stress in 30 degrees of flexion tests only the medial collateral ligament.

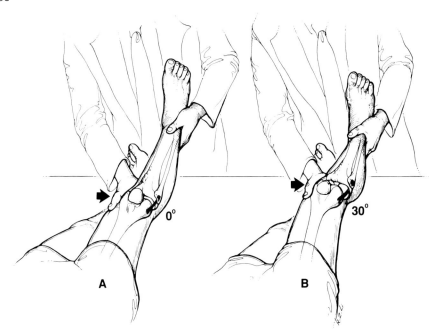

Fig. 3-13. The varus stress in extension tests the lateral collateral ligament and the posterolateral capsule. Stress in 30 degrees of flexion tests only the lateral collateral ligament.

There are a multitude of examinations for the integrity of the anterior cruciate ligament. The Lachman (Fig. 3-14) and anterior drawer tests (Fig. 3-15) apply anterior stress to the tibia at 30 and 90 degrees of flexion respectively. The Lachman is thought to be more sensitive for the posterolateral bundle of the cruciate, and the anterior drawer more sensitive for the anteromedial.

The flexion rotation drawer test builds on the Lachman test and notes tibial motion and femoral rotation from 15 degrees of flexion to 30 degrees (Fig. 3-16). Anterior force is applied to the tibia starting at 15 degrees of flexion. This leads to anterior subluxation much as in the Lachman test. With further knee flexion, the tibia reduces beneath the femur with a noticeable "clunk" and with noticeable internal rotation of the femur.

The jerk, pivot-shift, and Losee tests emphasize anterolateral motion of the tibia beneath the femur.

The jerk is initiated in flexion with associated internal tibial rotation and valgus stress (Fig. 3-17). This subluxes the lateral tibial condyle anteriorly. As the knee is brought into extension, the tibia reduces with a palpable "clunk," which is sometimes visible.

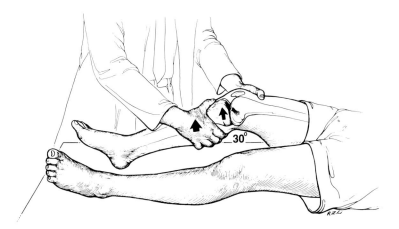

Fig. 3-14. The Lachman test is performed in 30 degrees of flexion with anterior force exerted on the proximal tibia.

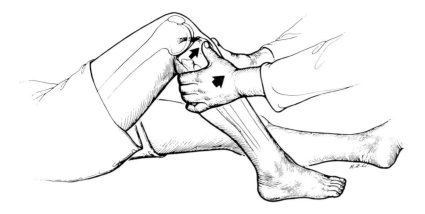

Fig. 3-15. The anterior drawer test is performed with the knee flexed to 90 degrees and with anterior force applied to the proximal tibia.

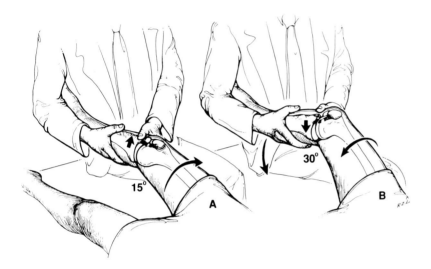

Fig. 3-16. The flexion rotation drawer test cradles the tibia in the examiner's hands and flexes the knee to demonstrate tibial reduction and internal femoral rotation.

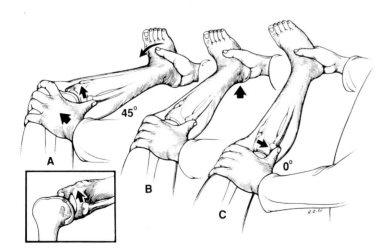

Fig. 3-17. The jerk test begins with the knee in flexion and applies internal rotation and valgus stress to demonstrate anterolateral subluxation of the tibia.

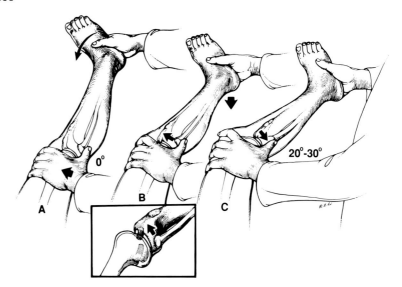

Fig. 3-18. The pivot-shift test begins with the knee in full extension and applies internal rotation and valgus stress to demonstrate anterolateral subluxation.

The pivot-shift test begins with the knee in full extension. Valgus stress is applied along with internal tibial rotation. As flexion is commenced, the lateral tibia again comes forward and then reduces with further flexion with a palpable "clunk" (Fig. 3-18). On occasion, this test may cause medial joint line pain indicative of an associated medial meniscal tear.

The Losee test is similar to the jerk test. It also begins with the knee in flexion and valgus stress. The tibia, however, is initially held in external rotation. As the knee is gradually extended, the tibia is internally rotated and the "clunk" of the reduction is again felt as in the jerk test. The test attempts to accentuate the subluxation with the external tibial rotation (Fig. 3-19).

The posterior cruciate can be evaluated with two primary tests and one secondary. The posterior Lachman is performed in 30 degrees of flexion, and the tibia is forced posteriorly (Fig. 3-20). The posterior drawer test (Fig. 3-21) positions the knee in 90 degrees of flexion and then applies the posterior force. The varus stress examination in full extension is said to include the posterior cruciate. From the discussion above, if the lateral aspect of the knee opens with varus stress in full extension, this includes the lateral collateral ligament and the posterolateral capsular structures. Some examiners believe that this opening cannot occur without posterior cruciate disruption. The authors disagree with this statement and believe that the varus stress examination can be positive with an intact posterior cruciate.

The posteromedial capsule is tested with the Slocum test (anterior drawer test with external rotation of the lower leg). When the tibia is externally rotated, the posteromedial capsule should tighten and allow less anterior excursion than the drawer test in neutral rotation. When the posteromedial capsule is torn, the Slocum test demonstrates an increase in the anterior motion of the tibia versus the drawer test in neutral, and the tibia tends to "roll out" (Fig. 3-22).

The posterolateral capsule is tested with the anterior drawer test in internal tibial rotation. If the posterolateral capsule is torn, the drawer test with internal rotation will show an increase in the anterior motion versus the drawer test in neutral, and the tibia will tend to "roll in" (Fig. 3-23). The hyperextension recurvatum sign correlates with injury to the posterolateral capsule. If the leg is held in full extension, the knee hyperextends, and the tibia exter-

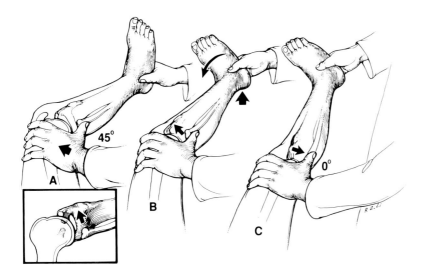

Fig. 3-19. The Losee test begins with the knee in flexion but externally rotates the foot. Valgus stress is applied and the tibia is internally rotated as the knee is extended.

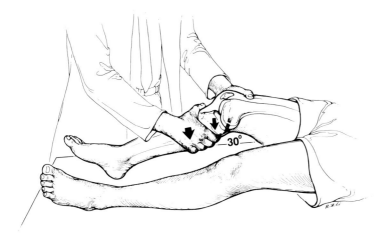

Fig. 3-20. The posterior Lachman test applies posterior force to the proximal tibia with the knee flexed 30 degrees.

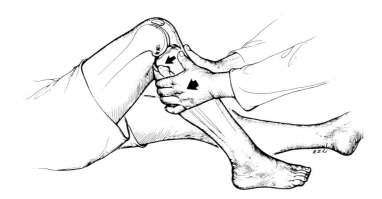

Fig. 3-21. The posterior drawer test is performed in 90 degrees of flexion with posterior force on the proximal tibia.

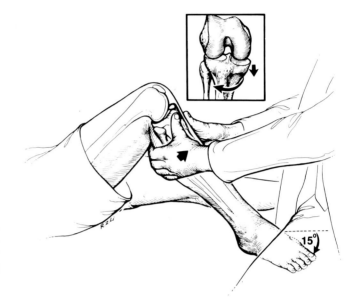

Fig. 3-22. The Slocum test is performed in 90 degrees of flexion with the foot externally rotated. Anterior proximal tibial force is applied to test the posteromedial capsule.

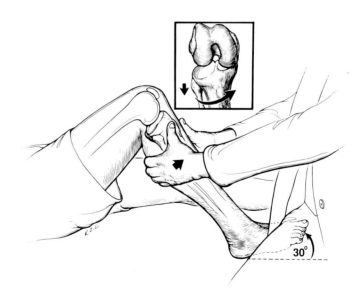

Fig. 3-23. The posterolateral capsule is tested with the knee flexed to 90 degrees. Anterior proximal tibial force is applied with the tibia internally rotated.

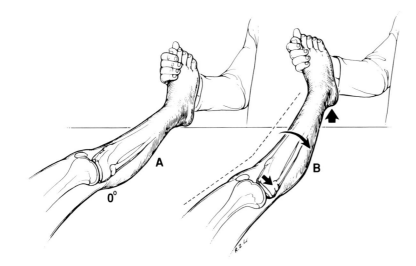

Fig. 3-24. The hyperextension recurvatum test demonstrates the increased extension of the knee along with the external tibial rotation and dropback.

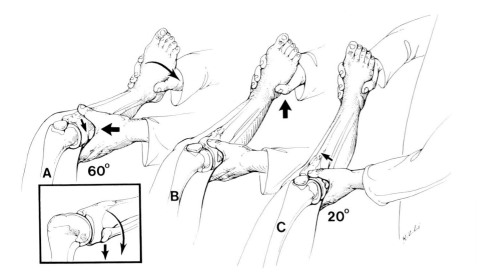

Fig. 3-25. The reverse pivot shift begins with the knee flexed and externally rotates the tibia. The knee is then extended and the posterolateral capsular laxity demonstrated.

nally rotates because of the absence of the posterolateral capsule and its supporting structures (Fig. 3-24). The reverse pivot shift test is performed with the tibia externally rotated and the knee flexed. As the knee is extended, the tibia reduces with a palpable clunk, indicating that the posterolateral capsule is deficient (Fig. 3-25).

Table 3-2 lists the stress tests in the order of their sensitivity.

Table 3-2. Stress Examination (In Order of Sensitivity)

Ligament/Capsule	Test
Medial collateral ligament	Valgus stress (30 degrees flexion)
Lateral collateral ligament	Varus stress (30 degrees flexion)
Anterior cruciate ligament	Lachman, flexion rotation drawer, anterior drawer, jerk, pivot, Losee
Posterior cruciate ligament	Posterior Lachman, posterior drawer, sag (late), (?varus laxity in full extension)
Posteromedial capsule	Valgus in full extension, Slocum
Posterolateral capsule	Varus in full extension, drawer in internal rotation, hyperextension recurvatum test

SUGGESTED READINGS

Apley AC: The diagnosis of meniscal injuries. J Bone Joint Surg 1947;29:78–84

Bargar WL, Moreland JR, Markolf KL, Shoemaker SC: The effect of tibia-foot rotatory position on the anterior drawer test. Clin Orthop 1983 Mar;(173):200–3

**Committee on the Medical Aspects of Sports, American Medical Association: Standard Nomenclature of Athletic Injuries, pp.99–101. American Medical Association, Chicago, 1968

Daniel DM, Stone ML, Barnett P, Sachs R: Use of the quadriceps active test to diagnose posterior cruciate-ligament disruption and measure posterior laxity of the knee. J Bone Joint Surg [Am] 1988 Mar;70(3):386–91

Feagin JA, Cooke TD: Prone examination for anterior cruciate ligament insufficiency. J Bone Joint Surg [Br] 1989 Nov;71(5):863

**Fetto JF, Marshall JL: Injury to the anterior cruciate ligament producing the pivot-shift sign. J Bone Joint Surg [Am] 1979 Jul;61A(5):710–4

*Galway RD, Beaupre A, MacIntosh DL: Pivot shift: A clinical sign of symptomatic anterior cruciate insufficiency. J Bone Joint Surg (Abstract) 1972;54B:763–764

**Hughston JC, Andrews JR, Cross MJ, Moschi A: Classification of knee ligament instabilities. Part I. The medial compartment and cruciate ligaments. J Bone Joint Surg [Am] 1976 Mar;58(2):159–72

**Hughston JC, Andrews JR, Cross MJ, Moschi A: Classification of knee ligament instabilities. Part II. The lateral compartment. J Bone Joint Surg [Am] 1976 Mar;58(2):173–9

Jakob RP, Hassler H, Staeubli HU: Observations on rotatory instability of the lateral compartment of the knee. Experimental studies on the functional anatomy and pathomechanics of the true and the reversed pivot shift sign. Acta Orthop Scand 1981;52(supplement 191):1–32

Larson RL: Physical examination in the diagnosis of rotatory instability. Clin Orthop 1983 Jan-Feb;(172):38–44

*Losee RE: Diagnosis of chronic injury to the anterior cruciate ligament. Orthop Clin North Am 1985 Jan;16(1):83–97

Losee RE, Johnson TR, Southwick WO: Anterior subluxation of the lateral tibial plateau. J Bone Joint Surg 1978;60A:1015–1030

*McMurray TP: The semilunar cartilages. Br J Surg 1942;29:407–414

Marshall JL, Baugher WH: Stability examination of the knee: a simple anatomic approach. Clin Orthop 1980 Jan-Feb;(146):78–83

*Noyes FR, Butler D, Grood E, et al: Clinical paradoxes of anterior cruciate instability and a new test to detect its instability. Orthop Trans 1978;2:36–37

Slocum DB, Larson RL: Rotatory instability of the knee. Its pathogenesis and a clinical test to demonstrate its presence. J Bone Joint Surg 1968;50A:211–225

*Torg JS, Conrad W, Kalen V: Clinical diagnosis of anterior cruciate ligament instability in the athlete. Am J Sports Med 1976;4:84–93

** Source reference
* Reference of major interest

Roentgenographic Techniques

4

The initial roentgenographic evaluation of the knee includes four standard views: anteroposterior (AP), preferably standing (Fig. 4-1); lateral (Fig. 4-2); notch or tunnel view (AP with the knee flexed 30 degrees, allowing the beam to pass through the knee without the patellar shadow overlying the intercondylar notch) (Fig. 4-3); and a Hughston skyline view (Fig. 4-4).

The standard non-weight-bearing AP view shows the tibiofemoral surfaces but cannot include a measurement of alignment because the element of gravity is eliminated. Therefore, the erect film allows one to evaluate the joint surfaces and determine alignment at the same time.

With the appropriate roentgenogram, one can then determine either the anatomic alignment of the limb (using the medullary canal of the femur and the tibia as reference) or the mechanical alignment (using the femoral head, joint line of the knee, and the center of the talus) (Fig. 4-5).

Recent publications indicate that the weight-bearing study with a PA projection and the knee flexed 15 degrees allows better definition of arthritic changes. While this may very well be true, the view should not be substituted for the traditional views to establish alignment of the limb.

A true lateral roentgenogram reveals the notch on the lateral femoral condyle and the larger medial condyle and shows the sulcus area of the lateral condyle projecting more anterior than that of the medial condyle. The medial tibial plateau projects both anterior and posterior to the lateral tibial plateau, and the medial concavity can be distinguished from the lateral convexity (Fig. 4-2).

The notch view reveals any early arthritic encroachment, possible loose bodies, or cruciate disruption with bone involvement on either the tibial or femoral side (Fig. 4-6).

There are a multitude of skyline views for the patellofemoral joint. They are all an attempt to evaluate the articular surfaces and the alignment of the patella with the anterior sulcus of the femur. The critical area for patellar tracking and alignment is in the first 30 degrees from full extension into flexion. The views completed in this range of motion can demonstrate the relationship of the patella with the sulcus and measure alignment. Unfortunately, it is difficult for patients to cooperate during the examination and for technicians to complete the study. The views of Furmaier, Knutsson, Laurin, and Merchant are examples of such alignment roentgenograms (Fig. 4-7).

Skyline films completed with the knee flexed beyond 45 degrees can only be utilized to examine the surfaces. As flexion occurs, the patella centralizes in the femoral sulcus and the patellar surface contact shifts to the medial and lateral facets. Beyond 40 degrees of flexion, patellar subluxation and/or dislocation may be completely overlooked. However, because the views are easily completed, they represent the most common skyline roentgenograms of the knee. Hughston and Settegast are two of the more common skyline views (Fig. 4-8).

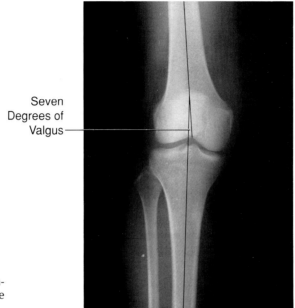

Seven
Degrees of
Valgus

Fig. 4-1. Anteroposterior roentgen-ogram of the right knee in the weight-bearing position.

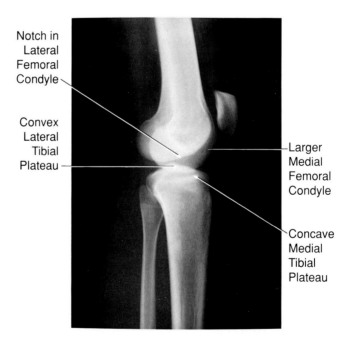

Notch in
Lateral
Femoral
Condyle

Convex
Lateral
Tibial
Plateau

Larger
Medial
Femoral
Condyle

Concave
Medial
Tibial
Plateau

Fig. 4-2. Lateral roentgenogram of the knee.

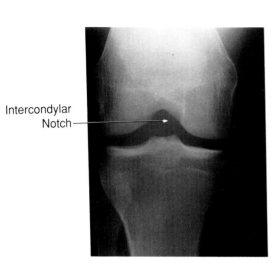

Intercondylar Notch

Fig. 4-3. Tunnel roentgenogram of the knee.

Medial Femoral Condyle

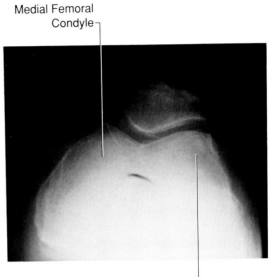

Lateral Femoral Condyle

Fig. 4-4. Hughston skyline view of the knee.

Anatomic Axis   Mechanical Axis

7°   0°

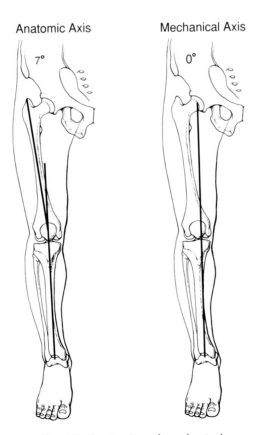

Fig. 4-5. Anatomic and mechanical alignment of the lower leg.

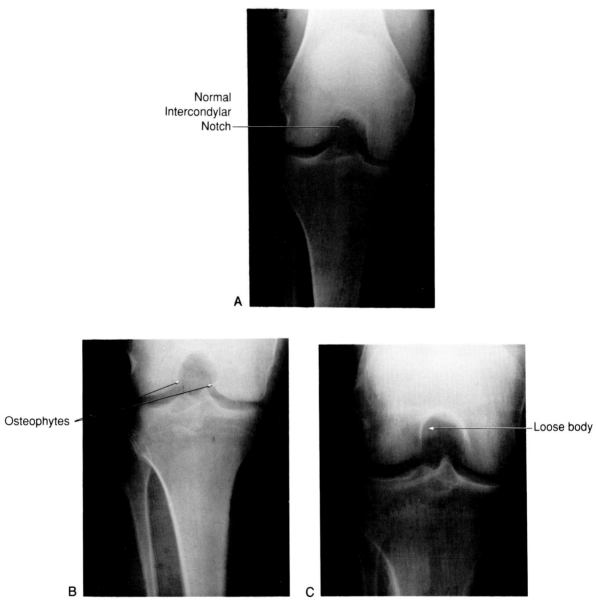

Fig. 4-6. Notch views demonstrating (A) the normal, (B) arthritic encroachment, and (C) intercondylar loose bodies.

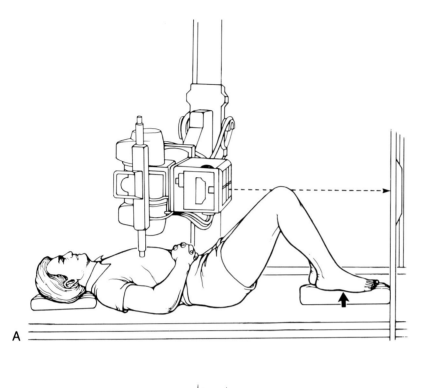

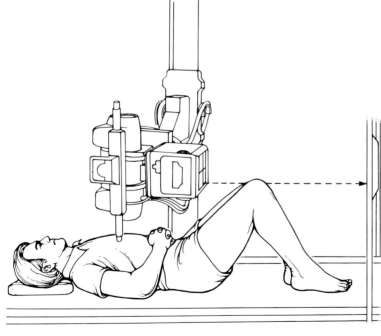

Fig. 4-7. (A) Furmaier's view is taken with the beam from head to foot and the feet slightly elevated from the table top. (B) Knutsson's view is taken with the beam from head to foot with the feet flat on the table top. (*Figure continues.*)

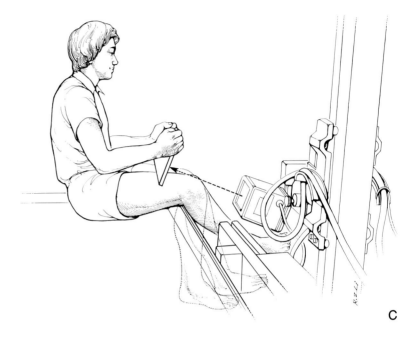

C

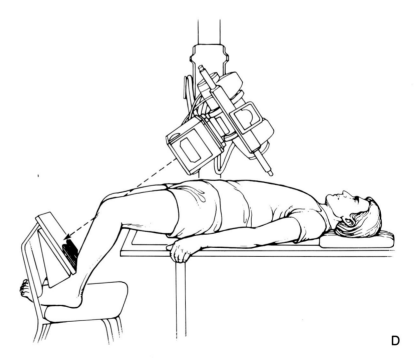

Fig. 4-7 *(Continued).* (C) Laurin's view is taken with the knees flexed 30 to 45 degrees and the beam from distal to proximal. (D) Merchant's view is taken with the knees flexed 30 to 45 degrees and the beam from proximal to distal.

D

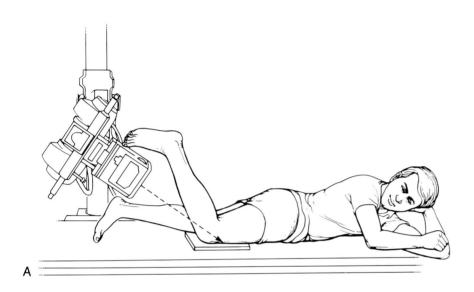

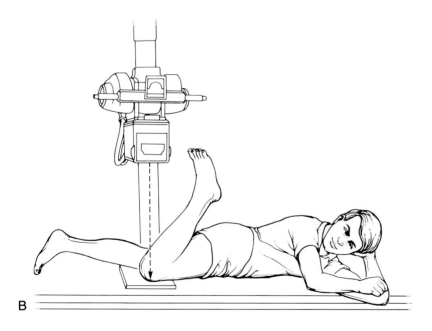

Fig. 4-8. (A) Hughston skyline view.
(B) Settegast skyline view.

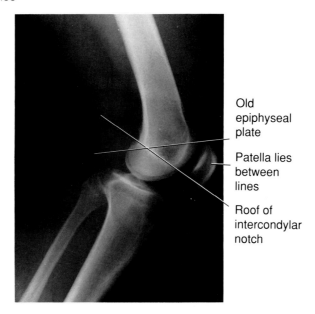

Old
epiphyseal
plate

Patella lies
between
lines

Roof of
intercondylar
notch

Fig. 4-9. Lateral view of the knee with Blumensaat's lines illustrating normal height of the patella.

Some of the roentgenographic views have been examined for the possibility of using measurements or ratios to develop normal standards. Blumensaat evaluated the lateral view (with the knee flexed 30 degrees) for patellar height and described lines along the old distal femoral epiphysis and across the roof of the intercondylar notch. If the patella was positioned in this area, then it was normal; if the patella was above these lines, it was considered to be high-riding (Fig. 4-9). Insall and Salvati used a ratio of the patellar tendon length on the lateral roentgenogram (with the knee flexed 30 degrees) to the oblique patellar length (Fig. 4-10A). They considered a ratio of 1.0 to 1.2 to be normal. A higher ratio indicates patella alta. Blackburne and Peel, using the lateral roentgenogram with at least 30 degrees of flexion, measured the patellar articular surface length and compared it to the height above the tibial plateau line. Their normal ratio was 0.54 to 1.06 (Fig. 4-10B). Merchant and Laurin developed measurements for their views using the sulcus of the femur and the facets of the patella to standardize the patellar position (Fig. 4-11). Jacobsen published an entire supplement on stress roentgenographic measurements to evaluate ligamentous injuries, and Tria applied a ratio technique for medial knee disruptions (Fig. 4-12).

MAGNETIC RESONANCE IMAGING

Nuclear magnetic resonance imaging (MRI) is best applied to the soft tissue structures of the knee. It is most accurate for the menisci and then for the collateral and the posterior cruciate ligaments, followed by knee effusions, the anterior cruciate ligament, and then Baker's cysts and ganglia, in that order. On occasion the medullary canal of the femur and the tibia can be visualized for the presence of avascular necrosis or other medullary tumorous conditions (Fig. 4-13).

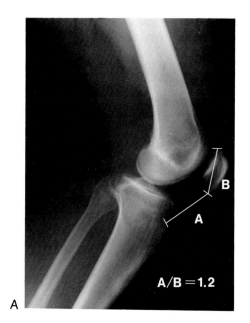

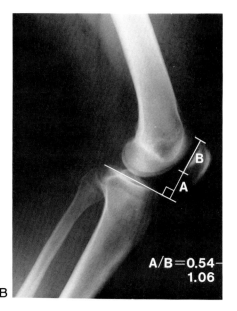

Fig. 4-10. (A) Lateral view of the knee with the Insall-Salvati ratio lines drawn indicating a normal ratio of 1.2 (patellar tendon to the patellar length). (B) Lateral view of the knee with the Blackburne and Peele measurements drawn indicating a normal ratio (height above the tibial plateau line [A] divided by the patellar articular surface length [B]) of 0.84.

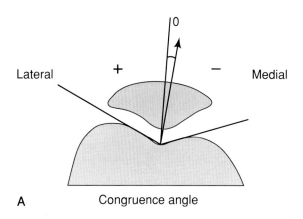

A   Congruence angle

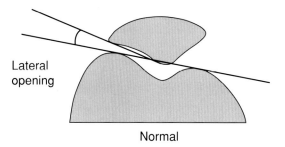

Lateral opening

Normal

Lateral   Medial

Fig. 4-11. (A) The Merchant view measures the sulcus angle of the femur and bisects it. The lowest point of the patella is then marked and the angle formed by that line with the bisecting line is the congruence angle. (B) The Laurin view relates a line across the femoral condyles to a line along the lateral patellar facet. Normal alignment leads to an angle opening laterally, and abnormal alignment leads to a medially opening angle.

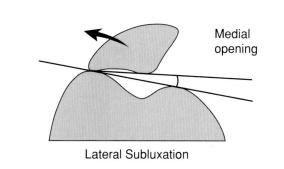

B   Lateral Subluxation

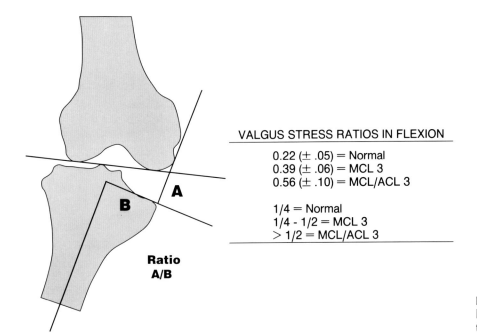

VALGUS STRESS RATIOS IN FLEXION

0.22 (± .05) = Normal
0.39 (± .06) = MCL 3
0.56 (± .10) = MCL/ACL 3

1/4 = Normal
1/4 - 1/2 = MCL 3
> 1/2 = MCL/ACL 3

Ratio
A/B

Fig. 4-12. The triad ratio for medial knee injuries incorporates a ratio for the medial opening.

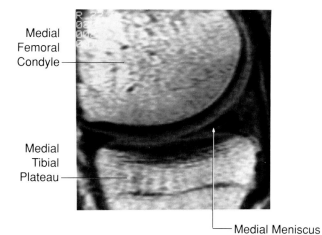

Medial Femoral Condyle

Medial Tibial Plateau

Medial Meniscus Tear

Fig. 4-13. Magnetic resonance imaging sagittal view of a torn posterior horn of the medial meniscus.

ARTHROGRAMS

The single and double contrast arthrograms have essentially been replaced by MRI. Rarely, the arthrogram may be more helpful in visualizing a Baker's cyst by causing it to distend more during the course of the actual examination (Fig. 4-14).

COMPUTERIZED TOMOGRAPHY

Computerized tomography (CT) scans are best for visualizing the bone structures of the knee. They may be employed to visualize articular surfaces in tibial plateau fractures and may be somewhat helpful for the patellofemoral articulation (Fig. 4-15); however, MRI is almost as accurate and does not involve x-ray exposure. Salter-Harris fractures can be visualized clearly with this technique and the adequacy of a reduction thoroughly reviewed.

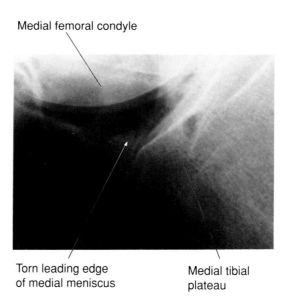

Medial femoral condyle

Torn leading edge of medial meniscus

Medial tibial plateau

Fig. 4-14. Arthrogram demonstrating a torn medial meniscus.

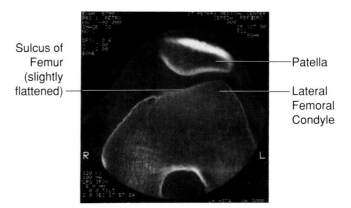

Sulcus of Femur (slightly flattened)

Patella

Lateral Femoral Condyle

Fig. 4-15. Computed tomographic scan of the patellofemoral joint illustrating lateral patellar subluxation.

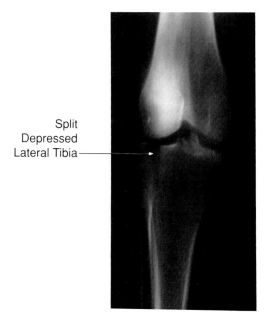

Split
Depressed
Lateral Tibia———

Fig. 4-16. Tomogram of a depressed-split tibial plateau fracture.

SPECIALIZED STUDIES

Roentgenographic tomograms are sometimes useful in the evaluation of the articular surfaces. Millimeters of depression are important and may decide whether surgical intervention is indicated (Fig. 4-16). CT scans are probably more accurate, especially if they are reconstructed three-dimensionally; however, CT scans involve more x-ray exposure and are not readily available in most centers.

SCINTIGRAPHIC TECHNIQUES

Technetium monosulfate scans are useful for the evaluation of tumors, fractures, avascular necrosis, and joint replacements. Both the early and late phases are integral parts of the study. Increased early flow correlates with a synovitis, which then requires further diagnostic testing to explain its etiology. The late flow pattern must be characterized both for its intensity and its location in the knee (Fig. 4-17).

Gallium sulfate scanning is an integral part of the evaluation for infection. The images from the study must be compared with the technetium scans and visually differentiated to determine which of the two illustrates greater uptake. Some centers have tried to use computers to average the uptake and compare the two. The latter approach has not found strong support (Fig. 4-18).

Indium-111 white cell tagged scans are more specific for infectious processes but are not routinely done by most nuclear medicine departments because of availability and additional expense (Fig. 4-19).

Right Knee
with "Cold
Spot" from
Knee
Replacement

Left Knee with
Diffuse Uptake

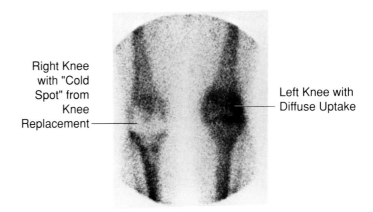

Fig. 4-17. Technetium scan of a normal right total knee arthroplasty and an arthritic left knee.

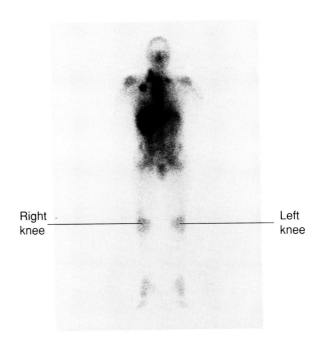

Right
knee

Left
knee

Fig. 4-18. A normal gallium scan of both knees.

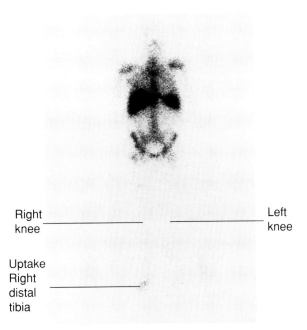

Right knee _____   _____ Left knee

Uptake
Right
distal _____
tibia

Fig. 4-19. A normal indium scan of the knees with osteomyelitis involving the right distal tibia.

SUGGESTED READINGS

*Blackburne JS, Peel TE: A new method of measuring patellar height. J Bone Joint Surg [Br] 1977 May;59(2):241–2

Blumensaat C: Die lageabweichungen and verrenkungen der kniescheibe. Ergebn Chir Orthop 1938;31:149–223

Cockshott WP, Racoveanu NT, Burrows DA, Ferrier M: Use of radiographic projections of knee. Skeletal Radiol 1985;13(2):131–3

Dalinka MK, Garofola J: The infrapatellar synovial fold: a cause for confusion in the evaluation of the anterior cruciate ligament. Am J Roentgenol 1976 Oct;127(4):589–91

*Freiberger RH, Pavlov H: Knee arthrography. Radiology 1988 Feb;166(2):489–92

Ghelman B: Meniscal tears of the knee: evaluation by high-resolution CT combined with arthrography. Radiology 1985 Oct;157(1):23–7

Glashow JL, Katz R, Schneider M, Scott WN: Double-blind assessment of the value of magnetic resonance imaging in the diagnosis of anterior cruciate and meniscal lesions. J Bone Joint Surg [Am] 1989 Jan;71(1):113–9

Hunter JC, Hattner RS, Murray WR, Genant HK: Loosening of the total knee arthroplasty: detection by radionuclide bone scanning. AJR 1980 Jul;135(1):131–6

Inoue M, Shino K, Hirose H et al: Subluxation of the patella. Computed tomography analysis of patellofemoral congruence. J Bone Joint Surg [Am] 1988 Oct;70(9):1331–7

*Insall J, Salvati E: Patella position in the normal knee joint. Radiology 1971;101:101–104

Iversen BF, Sturup J, Jacobsen K, Andersen J: Implications of muscular defense in testing for the anterior drawer sign in the knee. A stress radiographic investigation. Am J Sports Med 1989 May-Jun;17(3):409–13

Jacobsen K: Stress radiographical measurement of the anteroposterior, medial and lateral stability of the knee joint. Acta Orthop Scand 1976 Jun;47(3):335–4

**Jacobsen K: Gonylaxometry. Stress radiographic measurement of passive stability in the knee joints of normal subjects and patients with ligament injuries. Accuracy and range of application. Acta Orthop Scand Suppl 1981;52(194):1–263

Kaye JJ: Knee arthrography today. Radiology 1985 Oct;157(1):265–6

** Source reference
* Reference of major interest

Kujala UM, Osterman K, Kormano M et al: Patellar motion analyzed by magnetic resonance imaging. Acta Orthop Scand 1989 Feb;60(1):13–6

*Laurin CA, Dussault R, Levesque HP: The tangential x-ray investigation of the patellofemoral joint: x-ray technique, diagnostic criteria and their interpretation. Clin Orthop 1979 Oct;(144):16–26

McPhee IB, Fraser JG: Stress radiology in acute ligmentous injuries of the knee. Injury 1980;12:383–388

*Merchant AC, Mercer RL, Jacobsen RH: Roentgenographic analysis of patellofemoral congruence. J Bone Joint Surg 1974;56:1391–1396

Mooar P, Gregg J, Jacobstein J: Radionuclide imaging in internal derangements of the knee. Am J Sports Med 1987 Mar-Apr;15(2):132–7

Passariello R, Trecco F, De Paulis F et al: Computed tomography of the knee joint: technique of study and normal anatomy. J Comput Assist Tomogr 1983 Dec;7(6):1035–42

Reider B, Clancy W Jr, Langer LO: Diagnosis of cruciate ligament injury using single contrast arthrography. Am J Sports Med 1984 Nov-Dec;12(6):451–4

Rozing PM, Bohne WH, Insall J: Bone scanning for the evaluation of knee prosthesis. Acta Orthop Scand 1982 Apr;53(2):291–4

Tria AJ Jr, Geppert MJ, McBride M et al: The triad ratio: A roentgenographic ratio for medial knee injuries. Am J Knee Surgery 1990;3(3)126–130

Wetzner SM, Bezreh JS, Scott RD et al: Bone scanning in the assessment of patellar viability following knee replacement. Clin Orthop 1985 Oct;(199):215–9

Surgical Approaches 5

With the dawn of arthroscopy in Japan in the late sixties, the surgical approaches to the knee subsequently had to be divided into those requiring an arthrotomy and those requiring arthroscopy. As the science of arthroscopy has advanced and the technical support has improved, the incidence of arthroscopic procedures has increased and arthrotomies have become less and less frequent. It should be emphasized that arthrotomy of the knee is by no means outdated and often is the primary and only surgical solution. This discussion will consider arthrotomy first and then arthroscopy.

ARTHROTOMY OF THE KNEE

When discussing approaches to any joint, one must consider both the skin incision and the underlying arthrotomy. Many approaches will utilize similar skin incisions and yet have a completely different arthrotomy.

Medial Approaches

The median parapatellar (Langenbeck) incision begins along the medial aspect of the quadriceps tendon, skirts along the side of the patella, and then returns to the medial side of the patellar ligament as it proceeds distally. The arthrotomy enters the joint similarly on the medial aspect of the joint.

The Cave incision is hockey stick in shape with the transverse portion along the medial joint line and the stick portion ascending posteriorly. One could then enter the joint either anterior or posterior to the medial collateral ligament. Hoppenfeld and Deboer described a medial incision opposite to the Cave approach with the concave portion facing posterior. The vertical posteromedial incision (Henderson) is made behind the medial collateral ligament and affords the best exposure to the posterior aspect of the medial meniscus and the posteromedial aspect of the knee (Fig. 5-1).

Anterior Approaches

The midline incision made popular by Insall affords the best exposure to the majority of the knee. This is a modification of the Jones and Brackett midline incision that also included a patellar osteotomy for the arthrotomy. Insall utilized a median parapatellar arthrotomy after making the midline incision.

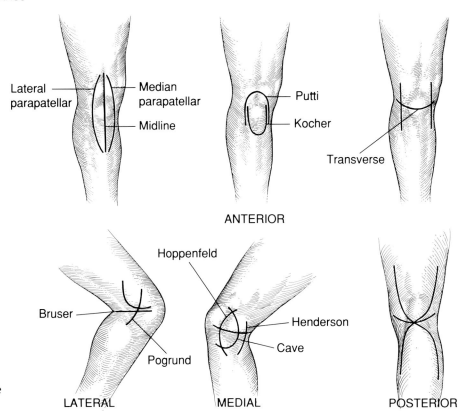

Fig. 5-1. The incisions of the knee joint.

Coonse and Adams described a median parapatellar incision and then a quadriceps turn down to enter the joint (Fig. 5-2). Insall described a modification of this with a long oblique incision across the quadriceps tendon with the base lateral and then a turn down (Fig. 5-3). Others have used the same midline skin incision and then elevated the tibial tubercle to expose the joint (Fig. 5-4).

The Kocher U incision and Putti inverted U have both become obsolete, primarily because of the complications secondary to the compromise of the blood supply to the surrounding skin (Fig. 5-1).

The transverse incision is cosmetically pleasing but does not permit extensile exposure. The approach also presents a skin healing problem if a vertical incision becomes necessary at a later time.

Lateral Approaches

The lateral parapatellar incision (Kocher) is seldom used in knee surgery but should be included for completeness. The Kocher incision may be helpful when one is considering a lateral joint surgery such as a unicompartmental replacement or total replacement in the valgus aligned knee. The horizontal lateral incision (Bruser) was commonly used to approach the lateral meniscus. With the knee flexed to 90 degrees, the iliotibial band was incised in the line of its fibers and then the capsule was opened anterior to the lateral collateral ligament. Brown modified the Bruser approach with knee flexion and a vertical incision anterior to the iliotibial band. Pogrund used an oblique incision from anterior to posterior and then flexed the knee to move the fat pad anteriorly (Fig. 5-1).

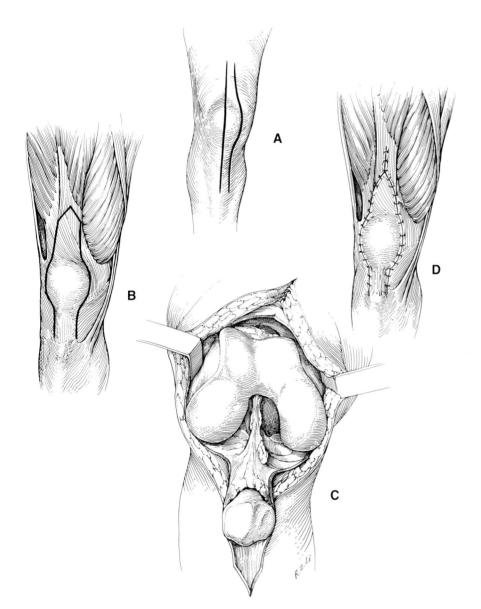

Fig. 5-2. The Coonse and Adams quadricepsplasty.

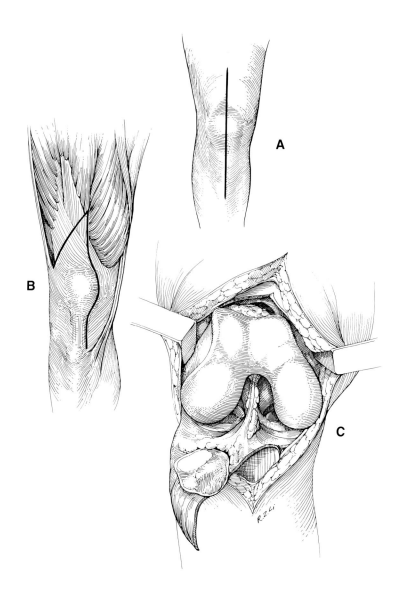

Fig. 5-3. The Insall quadriceps-plasty.

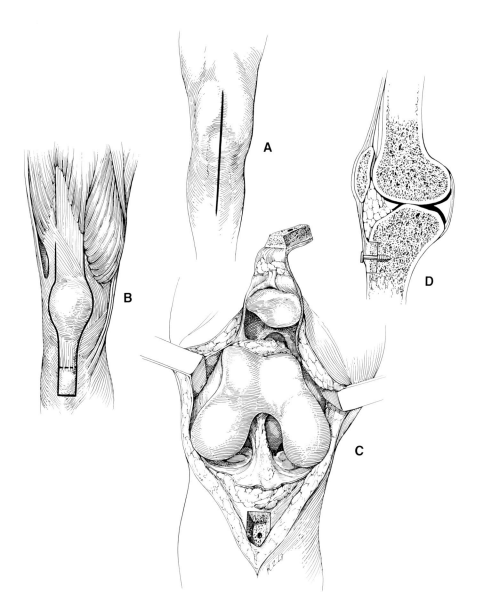

Fig. 5-4. Osteotomy of the tibial tubercle for knee joint exposure.

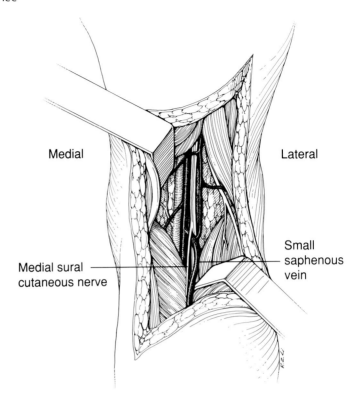

Fig. 5-5. The medial sural cutaneous nerve and the small saphenous vein are key landmarks for the approach to the posterior aspect of the knee.

Medial

Lateral

Medial sural cutaneous nerve

Small saphenous vein

Posterior Approaches

The popliteal space is a flexion crease and should not be crossed by a vertical incision, which would cause skin contractures. Therefore, the common incisions are either S-shaped or transverse within the flexion crease (Fig. 5-1).

The medial sural cutaneous nerve (posterior cutaneous nerve of the calf) and the small saphenous vein (lateral to the nerve) can be located in the subcutaneous tissue above the fascia. They form the key to the posterior exposure; the fascia should be incised lateral to them. The nerve is traced proximally to its origin from the tibial nerve, and the vein is traced to the popliteal vein (Fig. 5-5). This then allows the accurate exposure of the complete space with the nerve, vein, and artery in that order from superficial to deep at the level of the popliteal space.

ARTHROSCOPY OF THE KNEE

Arthroscopy began to develop an influence in this country in the early 1970s. It became much more popular with the addition of photographic supports through the early years. Now with the small microchip cameras that can be sterilized for use in the operative field and with small instruments that have a low breakage rate, the approach is well established.

There are five basic operative portholes. The inferomedial and inferolateral are the primary entries. The femoral condyle, tibial plateau surface, and the patellar ligament form the medial and lateral triangles. The arthroscope and the instruments are inserted through these sites. The mid-lateral and mid-

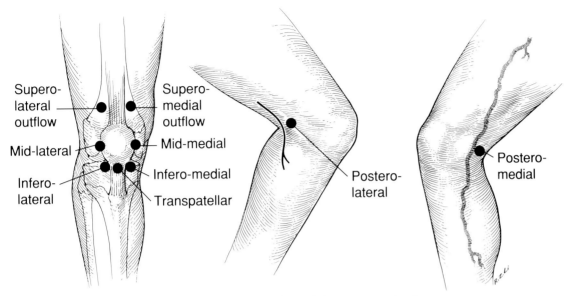

Fig. 5-6. The arthroscopic portholes and drainage sites for the knee.

medial punctures are sometimes of benefit for visualizing the anterior aspect of the joint. The transpatellar approach is sometimes of benefit in attempting to see directly into the posterior aspect of the knee through the intercondylar notch (Fig. 5-6). Most surgeons use a flow system with the inflow through the arthroscope and a drainage port-hole in the suprapatellar pouch.

SUGGESTED READINGS

**Abbott LC, Carpenter WF: Surgical approaches to the knee joint. J Bone Joint Surg 1945;27:277–310

Bruser DM: A direct lateral approach to the lateral compartment of the knee joint. J Bone Joint Surg [Br] 1960;42B:348–351

Cave EF: Combined anterior-posterior approach to the knee joint. J Bone Joint Surg 1935;17:427–430

Chambers GH: The prepatellar nerve: a cause of suboptimal results in knee arthrotomy. Clin Orthop 1972;82:157–159

Coonse KD, Adams JD: A new operative approach to the knee joint. Surg Gyn Obstet 1943;77:344–347

Fernandez DL: Anterior approach to the knee with osteotomy of the tibia tubercle for bicondylar tibial fractures. J Bone Joint Surg [Am] 1988 Feb;70(2):208–19

Hamberg P, Gillquist J, Lysholm J, Oberg B: The effect of diagnostic and operative arthroscopy and open meniscectomy on muscle strength in the thigh. Am J Sports Med 1983 Sep-Oct;11(5):289–92

**Hoppenfeld S, deBoer P: Surgical exposures in orthopaedics: the anatomic approach. JB Lippincott, Philadelphia, 1984

*Hughston JC: A surgical approach to the medial and posterior ligaments of the knee. Clin Orthop 1973 Mar-Apr;91:29–33

** Source reference
* Reference of major interest

Insall JN: A midline approach to the knee. J Bone Joint Surg 1971;53A:1584–1586

Jakob RP, Staubli HU, Zuber K, Esser M: The arthroscopic meniscal repair. Techniques and clinical experience. Am J Sports Med 1988 Mar-Apr;16(2):137–42

Medlar RC, Mandiberg JJ, Lyne ED: Meniscectomies in children. Report of long-term results (mean, 8.3 years) of 26 children. Am J Sports Med 1980 Mar-Apr;8(2):87–92

Miller DB Jr: Arthroscopic meniscus repair. Am J Sports Med 1988 Jul-Aug;16(4):315–20

Patel D: Proximal approaches to arthroscopic surgery of the knee. Am J Sports Med 1981 Sep-Oct;9(5):296–303

Pettrone FA: Meniscectomy: arthrotomy versus arthroscopy. Am J Sports Med 1982 Nov-Dec;10(6):355–9

Pogrund H: A practical approach for lateral meniscectomy. J Trauma 1976;16:365–367

Ligaments 6

This chapter will review ligamentous disruptions of the knee. Ligaments develop along with the menisci at about the forty-fifth day of gestation. At birth the ligaments have already developed into their adult form. Ligaments are the prime stabilizers of the joint. Loss of a ligament's integrity leads to changes in the mechanical balance of the joint. This may in turn cause injury to the menisci, joint surface changes, and subsequent arthritic degeneration.

CLINICAL PRESENTATION

Ligament tears are a result of an acute injury event. Often it is possible to obtain a history of the exact mechanism of injury, including the positioning of the joint at the time and any perception of tearing or a "pop." This information adds to the precision of the pretreatment diagnosis.

At the time of presentation, the injury is also classified as either acute (within 2 weeks of the episode) or chronic (beyond 2 weeks). Injuries to the medial and lateral collateral ligaments are best treated in the first 2 weeks. Cruciate ligament tears are sometimes treated slightly later in an attempt to avoid the associated acute joint reaction and possible loss of range of motion; however, this area remains controversial. If the injury is chronic, the approach may have to be altered because the tissues deteriorate and are not as easily repaired.

PHYSICAL EXAMINATION

Once the history has been obtained, a thorough examination should be completed with attention to both the ligaments and the associated capsular structures. Chapter 3 outlines the various tests that can be utilized to establish the integrity of each ligament and capsular area.

Disruption of the ligaments leads to specific instabilities in the knee. Anteromedial instability causes abnormal shift of the tibia beneath the femur with anterior excursion, external rotation, and medial opening. This laxity is caused by disruption of the medial collateral, the posterior oblique, and the medial capsular ligaments. On physical examination the Slocum test (anterior drawer in external rotation) is the most sensitive. In a similar fashion, one can explain anterolateral, posterolateral, and posteromedial rotary instabilities of the knee. Table 6-1 summarizes the instability patterns along with the disrupted structures and the clinical findings on physical examination.

Table 6-1. Rotary Instability of the Knee

Instability*	Anatomy Disrupted	Clinical Tests**
Anteromedial	Medial collateral ligament Medial capsular ligament Posterior oblique ligament	Slocum (anterior drawer in external rotation)
Anterolateral	Lateral capsular ligament Anterior cruciate ligament Arcuate ligament (?partial)	Pivot-shift, jerk, Losee Slocum (anterior drawer in internal rotation)
Posterolateral	Arcuate ligament complex Lateral capsular ligament Biceps tendon Posterior cruciate ligament	External rotation recurvatum sign Reverse pivot-shift
Posteromedial	Medial collateral ligament Medial capsular ligament Posterior oblique ligament Anterior cruciate ligament Semimembranosus tendon stretching	Posterior drawer (medial tibia rotates posteriorly)

* In order of frequency
** In order of sensitivity

The four rotary instabilities of the knee can be taken one step further to the combined instabilities. The most common combination is the anteromedial and anterolateral instability. The next is the anterolateral and posterolateral instability. The final is the anteromedial and posteromedial instability. Each of these combinations can be demonstrated on a thorough physical examination and appropriately treated as outlined below.

The extent of the ligament disruption is graded from I to III. A grade I injury leads to minor tearing of the ligament with tenderness at the palpable sites of origin or insertion, but there is no detectable ligament laxity. The grade II injury leads to incomplete tearing. The stress examination reveals laxity of the ligament, but there is a distinct end point to the test. The grade III injury is a complete disruption of the ligament, and the stress examination indicates gross laxity with no distinct end point to the tests.

The knee ligament laxity demonstrated on the physical examination is graded from I to IV. This is subjective but is an attempt to establish a baseline for comparison both with other examiner's findings and for evaluation of the post-treatment result. The grade I laxity correlates with a 1 to 2 mm excursion. The laxity increases up to 10 mm with the grade IV testing. There are machines such as the KT-1000 Knee Arthrometer (MEDtronic Corporation, San Diego, California) and the Genucom (Faro Medical Technologies, Inc., Montreal, Canada) available for these testings; however, their findings are not routinely reproducible.

GENERALIZED TREATMENT

Grade I and II injuries of the collateral ligaments can be treated with non-operative approaches unless there is significant associated intra-articular pathology (such as a torn meniscus or an osteochondral fracture). Grade I tears can be mobilized as soon as the pain and tenderness decrease enough to permit motion (approximately 10 days). No supportive devices are required for adequate healing. Grade II tears are usually held in their anatomic position with a brace that will allow early motion to avoid knee flexion contracture while the ligament heals. This treatment is from 4 to 6 weeks.

Grade III injuries must be divided into those that only involve the ligament and those that have an associated capsular tear. The isolated grade III can often be braced; however, an associated capsular tear usually requires operative repair to prevent the rotary instability (outlined in Table 6-1).

The cruciate ligaments usually tear in an all-or-nothing way, and their treatment is determined by the degree of laxity (grade I to IV) on physical examination, the associated intra-articular pathology, the level of activity of the patient, and the surgeon's experience.

Ligament tears are primarily an adult injury. Most of the same injuries in the immature patient lead to epiphyseal fractures rather than to ligament disruption. Thus, this discussion concerns primarily the mature adult knee.

MEDIAL COLLATERAL LIGAMENT TEARS

Clinical Presentation

Tear of the medial collateral ligament is usually the result of a valgus injury with or without a secured foot.

Diagnosis

The valgus stress examination in 30 degrees of flexion is the most sensitive test. Palpation may occasionally be helpful in attempting to discover the site on the femur or the tibia where the tear has occurred. Arthrograms are no longer the test of choice because of the discomfort associated with the study, possible phlebitis, the roentgenographic exposure, and the lack of specificity. When a complete tear is present, however, the arthrogram may show the site of the tear and the leakage of contrast out from beneath the ligament disruption. MRI is somewhat helpful because it can identify the site of the ligament tear. Roentgenographic stress tests are supportive but not diagnostic because they are difficult to standardize with either an absolute measurement or an internal ratio.

Pathology

Medial collateral ligament tears progress as the injury force increases. Initially, the ligament elongates and then reaches the point where complete tearing occurs. The tear can occur on the femoral side (65 percent incidence), the tibial side (25 percent incidence), or at the level of the joint line (10 percent incidence) (Fig. 6-1). On occasion the ligament can tear on both sides of the joint. Although this is unusual, it must always be considered to avoid missing the complete pathology.

Treatment

Treatment is determined by the extent of the ligament disruption and the capsular involvement. Grade I, II, and III tears that do not have associated injuries can be treated with protected range of motion for 2 to 6 weeks. The grade III tear that extends into the posteromedial capsule results in anteromedial instability and requires surgical repair. The joint line tears and the double tears are best treated with operative approaches.

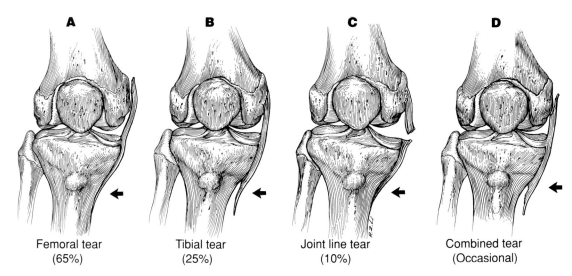

| A | B | C | D |
| Femoral tear (65%) | Tibial tear (25%) | Joint line tear (10%) | Combined tear (Occasional) |

Fig. 6-1. Medial collateral ligament tears occur most commonly on the femoral side. The tibial side is next, followed by the joint line. Tears on both sides do occur, but they are rather uncommon.

LATERAL COLLATERAL LIGAMENT TEARS

Clinical Presentation

Varus stress with internal rotation typically leads to lateral collateral ligament injuries. Lateral ligament tears are uncommon and are usually associated with other pathology in the posterolateral capsule and the posterior cruciate.

Diagnosis

The varus stress test in 30 degrees of flexion is the most specific for the lateral collateral ligament. Palpation may be helpful in establishing the site of the disruption. Plain roentgenograms may reveal a fibular head fracture. Because the ligament is essentially extra-articular, arthrograms are not particularly helpful. MRI may pinpoint the site of the tear. Once again, stress roentgenograms are supportive but not diagnostic.

Pathology

The majority of the lateral ligament tears occur on the fibular side (75 percent). Femoral tears are less common (20 percent), and midsubstance tears are rare (5 percent) (Fig. 6-2).

Treatment

The lateral collateral ligament is most commonly torn in association with the posterolateral capsule and the posterior cruciate. Disruption of the iliotibial band, the biceps femoris insertion into the fibular head, and the peroneal nerve are other associated injuries. The tear is usually approached through an arthrotomy and repaired in a primary fashion along with the other structures. Once appropriate repair has been completed, early protected motion is instituted.

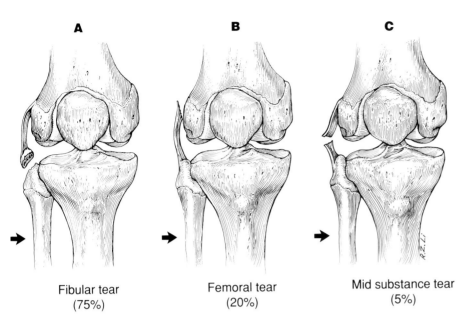

Fibular tear
(75%)

Femoral tear
(20%)

Mid substance tear
(5%)

Fig. 6-2. Lateral collateral ligament tears occur most commonly on the fibular side in association with a small bone fragment. The femoral side is next, followed by the mid substance tears.

ANTERIOR CRUCIATE LIGAMENT TEARS

Clinical Presentation

The anterior cruciate is usually injured in association with the medial collateral ligament as a part of the valgus stress leading to the triad of O'Donoghue. It can also be torn with a hyperextension force to the knee. With this mechanism of injury the anterior cruciate ligament is initially torn and then further hyperextension leads to meniscal tears, capsular tearing, posterior cruciate ligament disruption, and possible injury to the posterior neurovascular structures.

Diagnosis

Physical examination of the knee is still the best diagnostic approach for cruciate ligament injury. Chapter 3 lists the most sensitive tests for the anterior cruciate including the Lachman, flexion-rotation-drawer, anterior drawer, jerk, pivot-shift, and Losee (in the order of sensitivity). While arthrography did not prove to be very helpful, MRI is gradually improving and may eventually become diagnostic. Mechanical testing with devices such as the KT-1000 and the Genucom has also been useful but not diagnostic.

Pathology

Mid-substance tears of the anterior cruciate account for 75 percent of injuries; 20 percent are from the femoral attachment; and the remaining 5 percent are from the tibial side (Fig. 6-3). On occasion, the femoral or tibial disruptions may be associated with a periosteal sleeve or piece of bone. The

A   **B**   **C**

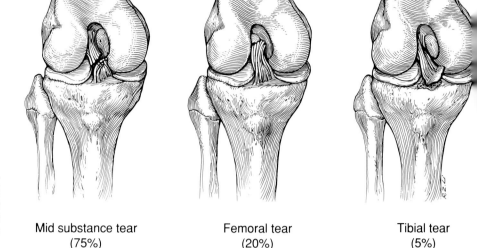

Fig. 6-3. The anterior cruciate ligament commonly tears in the mid substance; occasionally tears on the femoral side; and rarely tears on the tibial side (where a bone avulsion may occur).

Mid substance tear
(75%)

Femoral tear
(20%)

Tibial tear
(5%)

tibial bone fragment is smaller than the fragment seen with the tibial eminence fractures in children and should not be confused with that pathologic entity.

The ligament includes two bundles: anteromedial and posterolateral. Disruption of one bundle can sometimes occur. The anteromedial bundle is the smaller and weaker of the two. Loss of this segment leads to a positive anterior drawer test because the ligament is tighter in flexion and its absence is more noticeable in this position. The Lachman test may remain negative and the prognosis for the knee is fair to good.

Disruption of the stronger posterolateral bundle leads to a positive Lachman test because the segment is tightest as the knee moves into extension and the deficiency will be more prominent in that range of motion. The anterior drawer is usually slightly positive. Because the posterolateral bundle is the major portion of the anterior cruciate ligament, most surgeons equate its loss with complete ligament tearing.

Disruption of the synovial sleeve covering of the ligament has also been reported with subsequent compromise of one or both of the bundles because of loss of the vascularity from the middle geniculate. Some investigators do not believe that a partial tear can exist and maintain that injury to the synovium or one of the bundles ultimately leads to complete ligament compromise.

Treatment

The approach to treatment of the anterior cruciate ligament tear is fraught with controversy and emotion. A methodical evaluation should initially include a summary of the anatomy involved. The menisci, the remaining ligaments, the capsular structures, and articular surfaces (i.e., osteochondral fractures) should all be evaluated. Then, one must consider the patient's age, level of activity, and functional demands.

After full evaluation has been completed, the treatment options include immobilization with physical therapy and continued observation, arthroscopy with debridement of the torn cruciate and resection of any associated meniscal tears, primary ligament repair, primary ligament repair along with an intra-articular substitution, extra-articular substitution, or primary intra-articular reconstruction.

Because anterior cruciate ligament tears are associated with other pathology in 75 percent of injuries, observation is seldom a useful approach.

The surgical approaches range from simple arthroscopy to open arthrotomy and ligament reconstructions. The former procedure is best for the non-athletically demanding adult and the latter for the aggressive young athlete. At the present time, the better results are reported with arthroscopic ligament reconstructions; however, the findings are subject to individual experience and will certainly change with the progress presently occurring in the field today.

POSTERIOR CRUCIATE LIGAMENT TEARS

Clinical Presentation

The most common mechanism of injury is the dashboard or bumper blow to the anterior tibia with the knee flexed to 90 degrees. This results in posterior translation of the tibia beneath the femur and ligament tearing. The same injury is reproduced when an athlete falls directly upon the flexed knee striking the tibial tubercle against the ground with the foot plantar-flexed.

The second pattern of injury occurs at the extreme of hyperextension after the anterior cruciate and posterior capsule have given way and just before the neurovascular structures are torn.

Diagnosis

The posterior Lachman and the posterior drawer tests are the most sensitive for the posterior cruciate ligament. MRI often demonstrates the ligament clearly; however, its application in the clinical setting remains to be seen. As in the case of the anterior cruciate ligament, mechanical devices have not proven to be very valuable.

Pathology

Seventy percent of posterior cruciate ligament tears occur on the tibial side and are sometimes associated with a fleck of bone or even a larger fragment. Fifteen percent of the tears occur on the femoral side and another 15 percent occur in the mid substance (Fig. 6-4).

Treatment

As is the case in all of the ligament injuries, one must complete a thorough diagnostic evaluation of the knee first. If the ligament tear is an isolated injury in the midsubstance, the knee can often be treated with a short period of

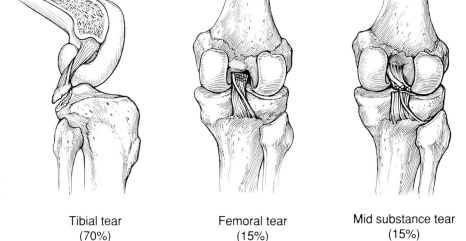

Fig. 6-4. The posterior cruciate ligament tears most commonly on the tibial side with an associated bone fragment. The femoral and mid substance tears are about equal in their occurrence.

Tibial tear
(70%)

Femoral tear
(15%)

Mid substance tear
(15%)

immobilization and then therapy. If the disruption is on the femoral or tibial side, surgical repair can be considered and often has excellent results if there is an associated bone fragment or periosteal sleeve. The main point concerning the posterior cruciate ligament is that the knee does surprisingly well without the ligament (even in the demanding athlete) if it is an isolated event; therefore, surgical intervention must be tempered by this consideration and only undertaken if the outcome is promising.

COMBINED LIGAMENT TEARS

Clinical Presentation

Combined ligament disruptions can be the result of a single plane injury taken to an extreme. The valgus stress initially tears the medial collateral ligament and continues on to tear the medial meniscus and then the anterior cruciate ligament. Multiple ligament injuries can also occur when a rotary motion is added to the single plane or when there is actually more than one direction of injury occurring sequentially.

Diagnosis

The same diagnostic techniques that are used to evaluate the individual ligaments should be used for the multiple evaluation. On occasion, one ligament injury may be overlooked when two or more ligaments are disrupted. Thoroughness is always essential. The difference between the two- and the three-ligament injury may be that the knee was dislocated. If dislocation has occurred, there is a high probability that there is an associated neurovascular injury (up to 50 percent incidence). This suspicion should lead the examiner to consider complete neurologic examination and possible femoral arteriogram to document the status of the popliteal artery before any surgical intervention is considered.

Pathology

The location of the ligament disruptions is less predictable when more than one tear has occurred; thus, patterns are not well established.

Treatment

When more than one ligament has been injured, the approach must be tempered by the pathology, age of the patient, demands of the patient, and the surgeon's experience.

The collateral ligaments should be given first priority with second importance given to the cruciates. Repairs should also be performed with the hope of instituting motion as early as possible to avoid loss of full range of motion.

SUGGESTED READINGS

American Medical Association, Committee on the Medical Aspects of Sports: Standard Nomenclature of Athletic Injuries. American Medical Association, Chicago, 1968, 99 – 101

*Arnoczky SP: Blood supply to the anterior cruciate ligament and supporting structures. Orthop Clin North Am 1985 Jan;16(1):15 – 28

**Arnoczky SP: Anatomy of the anterior cruciate ligament. Clin Orthop 1983 Jan-Feb;(172):19 – 25

Barber SD, Noyes FR, Mangine RE et al: Quantitative assessment of functional limitations in normal and anterior cruciate ligament-deficient knees. Clin Orthop 1990 Jun;(255):204 – 14

Bianchi M: Acute tears of the posterior cruciate ligament: clinical study and results of operative treatment in 27 cases. Am J Sports Med 1983 Sep-Oct;11(5):308 – 14

Carlson JM, French J: Knee orthoses for valgus protection. Experiments on 11 designs with related analyses of orthosis length and rigidity. Clin Orthop 1989 Oct;(247):175 – 92

Cawley PW, France EP, Paulos LE: Comparison of rehabilitative knee braces. A biomechanical investigation. Am J Sports Med 1989 Mar-Apr;17(2):141 – 6

Clancy WG Jr, Nelson DA, Reider B, Narechania RG: Anterior cruciate ligament reconstruction using one-third of the patellar ligament, augmented by extra-articular tendon transfers. J Bone Joint Surg [Am] 1982 Mar;64(3):352 – 9

Dahlstedt LJ, Dalen N: Knee laxity in cruciate ligament injury. Value of examination under anesthesia. Acta Orthop Scand 1989 Apr;60(2):181 – 4

*DeHaven KE: Diagnosis of acute knee injuries with hemarthrosis. Am J Sports Med 1980 Jan-Feb;8(1):9 – 14

DeLee JC, Curtis R: Anterior cruciate ligament insufficiency in children. Clin Orthop 1983 Jan-Feb;(172):112 – 8

Ellison AE: The pathogenesis and treatment of anterolateral rotatory instability. Clin Orthop 1980 Mar-Apr;(147):51 – 5

**Fetto JF, Marshall JL: The natural history and diagnosis of anterior cruciate ligament insufficiency. Clin Orthop 1980 Mar-Apr;(147):29 – 38

Fischer RA, Arms SW, Johnson RJ, Pope MH: The functional relationship of the posterior oblique ligament to the medial collateral ligament of the human knee. Am J Sports Med 1985 Nov-Dec;13(6):390–7

*Girgis FG, Marshall JL, Monajem A: The cruciate ligaments of the knee joint; Anatomical, functional, and experimental analysis. Clin Orthop 1975 Jan-Feb;(106):216–31

Goldman AB, Pavlov H, Rubenstein D: The Segond fracture of the proximal tibia: a small avulsion that reflects major ligamentous damage. AJR Am J Roentgenol 1988 Dec;151(6):1163–7

**Hughston JC, Andrews JR, Cross MJ, Moschi A: Classification of knee ligament instabilities. Part I. The medial compartment and the cruciate ligaments. J Bone Joint Surg [Am] 1976 Mar;58(2):159–72

**Hughston JC, Andrews JR, Cross MJ, Moschi A: Classification of knee ligament instabilities. Part II. The lateral compartment. J Bone Joint Surg [Am] 1976 Mar;58(2):173–9

*Jones KG: Results of use of the central one-third of the patellar ligament to compensate for anterior cruciate ligament deficiency. Clin Orthop 1980 Mar-Apr;(147):39–44

Jonsson H, Karrholm J, Elmqvist LG: Kinematics of active knee extension after tear of the anterior cruciate ligament. Am J Sports Med 1989 Nov-Dec;17(6):796–802

Kennedy JC, Hawkins RJ, Willis RB: Strain gauge analysis of knee ligaments. Clin Orthop 1977 Nov-Dec;(129):225–9

Marshall JL, Baugher WH: Stability examination of the knee: a simple anatomic approach. Clin Orthop 1980 Jan-Feb;(146):78–83

Marshall JL, Warren RF, Wickiewicz TL: Primary surgical treatment of anterior cruciate ligament lesions. Am J Sports Med 1982 Mar-Apr;10(2):103–7

**Marshall JL, Warren RF, Wickiewicz TL, Reider B: The anterior cruciate ligament: a technique of repair and reconstruction. Clin Orthop 1979 Sep;(143):97–106

Oliver JH, Coughlin LP: Objective knee evaluation using the Genucom Knee Analysis System. Clinical implications. Am J Sports Med 1987 Nov-Dec;15(6):571–8

Parolie JM, Bergfeld JA: Long-term results of nonoperative treatment of isolated posterior cruciate ligament injuries in the athlete. Am J Sports Med 1986 Jan-Feb;14(1):35–8

Reuben JD, Rovick JS, Schrager RJ et al: Three-dimensional dynamic motion analysis of the anterior cruciate ligament deficient knee joint. Am J Sports Med 1989 Jul-Aug;17(4):463–71

Tegner Y, Lysholm J: Rating systems in the evaluation of knee ligament injuries. Clin Orthop 1985 Sep;(198):43–9

Torg JS, Barton TM, Pavlov H, Stine R: Natural history of the posterior cruciate ligament-deficient knee. Clin Orthop 1989 Sep;(246):208–16

Tremblay GR, Laurin CA, Drovin G: The challenge of prosthetic cruciate ligament replacement. Clin Orthop 1980 Mar-Apr;(147):88–92

*Wojtys EM, Goldstein SA, Redfern M et al: A biomechanical evaluation of the Lenox Hill knee brace. Clin Orthop 1987 Jul;(220):179–84

Zoltan DJ, Reinecke C, Indelicato PA: Synthetic and allograft anterior cruciate ligament reconstruction. Clin Sports Med 1988 Oct;7(4):773–84

The Menisci   7

EMBRYOLOGY

The menisci are evident within the first 45 days of gestation (Fig. 7-1). They develop as blastemal cells connecting to the capsule and have the semi-lunar structure immediately. Thus, the discoid lateral meniscus is not a developmental abnormality but appears sometime after birth as part of an aberrant growth pattern.

The lateral meniscus develops slightly earlier than the medial.

ANATOMY

Chapter one reviews the basic anatomy of the menisci. Both are semicircular with the lateral slightly more C-shaped (Fig. 7-2). They are attached to the capsule about the periphery. The lateral meniscus attachment has a single defect where the popliteus tendon passes beneath the lateral collateral ligament from posteroinferior to anterosuperior to insert into the lateral femoral condyle (Fig. 7-3). In some cases the ligaments of Humphrey and Wrisberg may form attachments from the lateral meniscus to the medial femoral condyle, passing anterior and posterior to the posterior cruciate ligament (Fig. 7-4). The medial meniscus has no such ligamentous attachments.

The collagen fibers are oriented in two directions: radial and longitudinal (Fig. 7-5). This appears to give each meniscus greater mechanical strength to sustain both axial and rotational loading.

The blood supply is derived from branches of the geniculates. The vessels enter from the capsular attachment areas and penetrate inward (Fig. 7-6). The menisci do not derive any nourishment from the synovial fluid and, therefore, depend totally upon the peripheral vascular network for nourishment and healing. The body of the meniscus can be divided into three zones, with the inner one-third almost avascular (Fig. 7-7). The middle and outer thirds have better blood supply and show better healing properties if they are damaged.

The menisci have some normal variants that should not be confused with pathologic changes. The discoid meniscus (most commonly lateral) is circular in shape with just a slight central depression. It appears to develop sometime after birth (although this is somewhat debatable). If there is no tear in the discoid meniscus, then it is not considered to be abnormal.

The leading edge of the meniscus may occasionally present with an S wave pattern. If the body of the meniscus is stable to palpation, then this is not significant. In the knee with early arthritis, the leading edge may also be frayed, but this, again, is not pathologic.

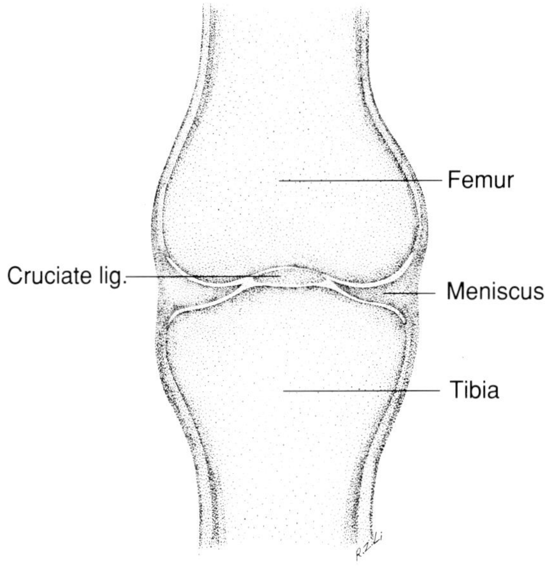

Fig. 7-1. The menisci can be distinguished within the first 45 days of gestation (From Hosea TM, Bechler J, Tria AJ: Embryology of the knee. In Scott WN: Ligament and Extensor Mechanism Injuries of the Knee: Diagnosis and Treatment. CV Mosby, St. Louis, 1991, with permission.)

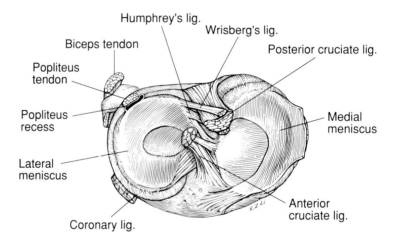

Fig. 7-2. Superior view of the right tibia illustrating the menisci and their relationship to the cruciates and the capsular structures.

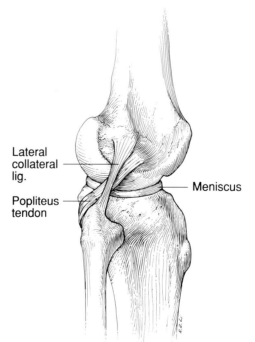

Fig. 7-3. The popliteus courses anteriorly beneath the lateral collateral ligament aside of the lateral meniscus.

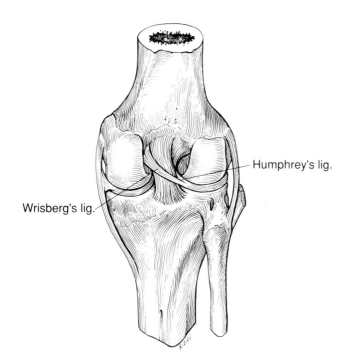

Humphrey's lig.

Wrisberg's lig.

Fig. 7-4. The ligaments of Humphrey and Wrisberg in relationship to the posterior cruciate ligament.

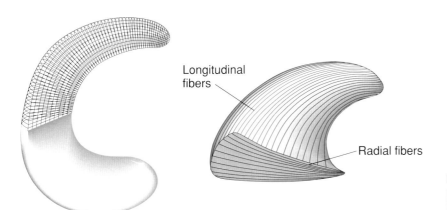

Longitudinal fibers

Radial fibers

Fig. 7-5. The collagen fibers of the meniscus are aligned radially and longitudinally.

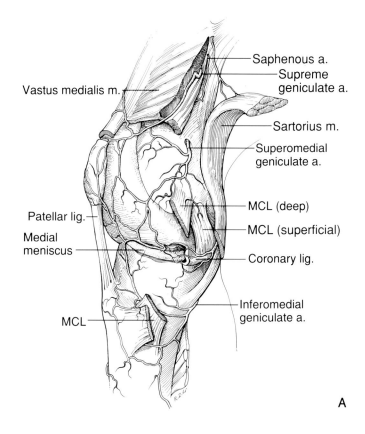

Saphenous a.

Supreme
geniculate a.

Vastus medialis m.

Sartorius m.

Superomedial
geniculate a.

MCL (deep)

Patellar lig.

MCL (superficial)

Medial
meniscus

Coronary lig.

MCL

Inferomedial
geniculate a.

A

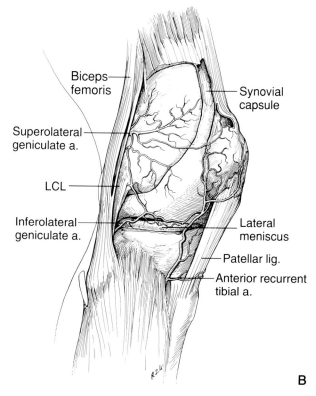

Biceps
femoris

Synovial
capsule

Superolateral
geniculate a.

LCL

Inferolateral
geniculate a.

Lateral
meniscus

Patellar lig.

Anterior recurrent
tibial a.

B

Fig. 7-6. (A) The medial meniscus blood supply enters from the periphery, predominantly from the inferomedial geniculate. (B) The lateral meniscus blood supply enters from the periphery, predominantly from the inferolateral geniculate.

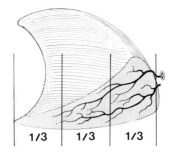

Fig. 7-7. The vascularity of the meniscus decreases as one progresses from the capsular attachment to the leading edge.

BIOMECHANICS

Motion of the knee causes motion of the menisci. The lateral meniscus moves anteroposteriorly more than the medial (Fig. 7-8). This may be related to the popliteus hiatus and the more lax capsular attachments or may reflect the lesser femorotibial joint congruity on the lateral side. The lateral tibial plateau is convex, and the lateral femoral condyle is notched and slightly flattened (Fig. 7-9).

The menisci also rotate as part of the screw-home mechanism. Despite the two degrees of motion (anteroposterior and internal/external rotation), the menisci still add to joint stability. Meniscectomy has been shown to increase rotary laxity.

The menisci increase the area of contact between the femoral condyle and the tibial plateau. Stress is defined as force divided by the area over which the force is applied. Thus, because the menisci increase the area, they decrease the stress across the joint.

At the same time, they are able to elongate circumferentially (to absorb hoop stresses) and do have some load-bearing potential.

The fibrocartilages aid in joint lubrication by decreasing the coefficient of friction. They aid in joint nutrition by compressing synovial fluid into the articular cartilage.

CLINICAL PRESENTATION

Tears of the menisci are either caused by an acute event or develop as a degenerative process. The history and age of the patient will certainly help in this respect. Younger patients tend to have injuries related to sports or trauma. Older patients tend to relate a gradual onset of the symptoms. These are only guidelines and one must always be aware of the unusual presentation.

Tears of the menisci lead to symptoms of pain and/or instability. The pain is usually aggravated by activities but may also be present at rest. The instability may lead to frank collapse of the joint or to a feeling of giving-way.

Acute ligament disruptions are often associated with meniscal tears. The knee with a chronic ligament imbalance may also develop a tear of the meniscus without further injury because of the abnormal joint motion. Thus, one must also keep in mind that a meniscus may be injured whenever a ligament injury is present.

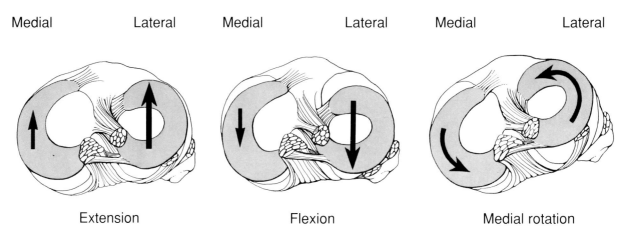

Medial   Lateral   Medial   Lateral   Medial   Lateral

Extension   Flexion   Medial rotation

Fig. 7-8. Despite the smaller anteroposterior width of the lateral tibial plateau, the lateral meniscus moves more than the medial through the range of motion of the knee.

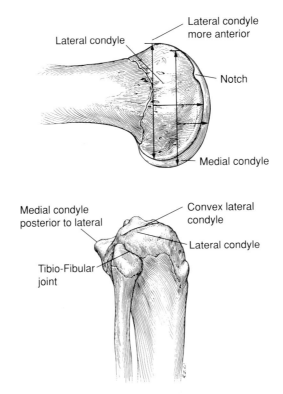

Lateral condyle more anterior

Lateral condyle

Notch

Medial condyle

Medial condyle posterior to lateral

Convex lateral condyle

Lateral condyle

Tibio-Fibular joint

Fig. 7-9. Lateral view of the distal femur and the proximal tibia showing the femoral notch and the convexity of the tibial plateau.

PHYSICAL EXAMINATION

The majority of the findings on the examination for the menisci center on the tenderness of the joint line, palpable clicks near the area of the tear, or rotational pain.

Table 3-1 summarizes the tests for meniscal tears and divides them up between the tests that depend upon a finding of direct tenderness versus a finding of pain with rotation of the joint. The majority of the examinations depend on rotation of the joint.

One may occasionally observe a cystic mass on the joint line. This most commonly indicates that the underlying meniscus has a tear that extends out to the peripheral attachment and the joint capsule.

ROENTGENOGRAPHIC TESTS

The initial evaluation of the knee is not complete without a full series of plain roentgenograms. The standard views are reviewed in Chapter 4. Failure to perform these studies before proceeding with further investigations can lead to major mistakes and complications. Tumors, fractures, and loose bodies are just some of the findings that are best evaluated with plain roentgenograms and might be overlooked with the use of other studies. The bone architecture must be thoroughly evaluated before turning to more sophisticated tests such as magnetic resonance imaging (MRI) and computerized tomography (CT).

Arthrograms of the knee (Fig. 7-10) were once very popular but are now essentially replaced by MRI (Fig. 7-11). These diagnostic studies are sometimes helpful in a difficult case but are not a necessary test in every evaluation. CT is excellent for bone detail but is not especially helpful for the menisci.

PATHOLOGY

Tears of the menisci can be categorized by their anatomic presentation. There is a horizontal or vertical component to every tear (Fig. 7-12). Each tear may extend partially across the body of the meniscus (incomplete tear) or completely across (complete tear). Along with the manner of tearing, there is also the gross anatomic appearance of the meniscus (Fig. 7-13).

The location of the tear is often predictable. Chronic tears and degenerative tears are associated with degradation of the fibrocartilage and proteoglycan disruption.

Over 70 percent of the tears occur in the posterior horns. This is thought to reflect the increased stresses in the posterior aspect of the knee with flexion.

The medial meniscal tears include the posterior flap, vertical longitudinal, bucket handle, and radial tears (in the order of incidence from the authors' experience) (Table 7-1 and Fig. 7-13).

The lateral tears include the radial, vertical longitudinal, bucket handle, and flap (in the order of incidence from the authors' experience) (Table 7-1 and Fig. 7-13).

Some of the tears are associated with cysts that herniate outside the capsule of the knee and are palpable on physical examination. One should take

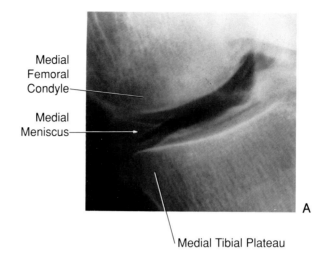

Medial
Femoral
Condyle

Medial
Meniscus

A

Medial Tibial Plateau

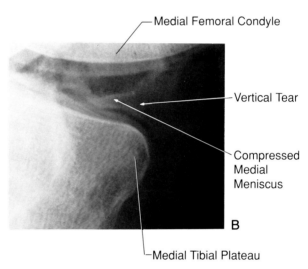

Medial Femoral Condyle

Vertical Tear

Compressed
Medial
Meniscus

B

Medial Tibial Plateau

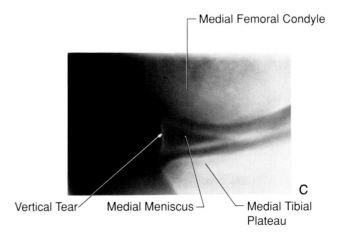

Medial Femoral Condyle

Vertical Tear   Medial Meniscus   Medial Tibial
Plateau

C

Fig. 7-10. Arthrograms illustrating (A) a normal medial meniscus; (B) a truncated (compressed) medial meniscus with a vertical tear; (C) a medial meniscus with a peripheral vertical tear.

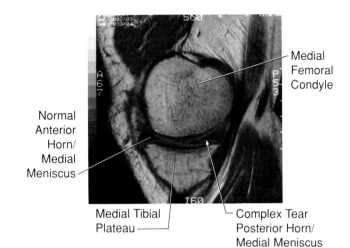

Medial
Femoral
Condyle

Normal
Anterior
Horn/
Medial
Meniscus

Medial Tibial
Plateau

Complex Tear
Posterior Horn/
Medial Meniscus

Fig. 7-11. MRI of the right knee illustrating a posterior horn tear of the medial meniscus.

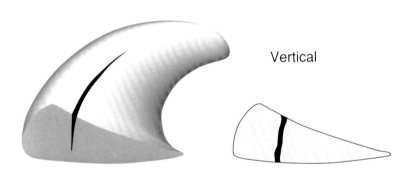

Vertical

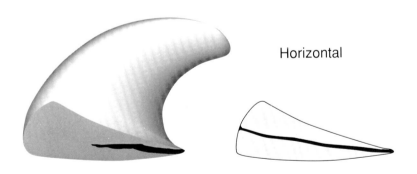

Horizontal

Fig. 7-12. The standard vertical and horizontal tears of the meniscus.

Incomplete

Complete

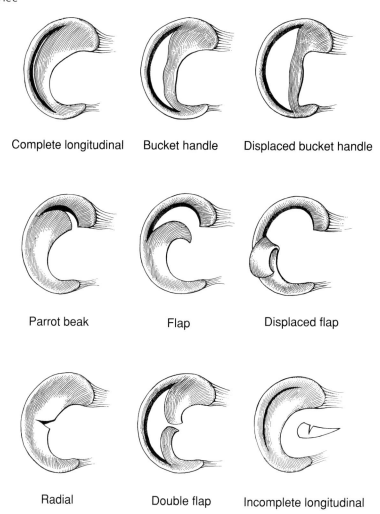

Complete longitudinal   Bucket handle   Displaced bucket handle

Parrot beak   Flap   Displaced flap

Radial   Double flap   Incomplete longitudinal

Fig. 7-13. The gross anatomic appearance of the common meniscal tears of the knee.

note of such masses because they are diagnostic of a tear and often save the patient further costly tests (Fig. 7-14). Degenerative tears, including cleavages and combinations, tend to be more complex.

THERAPY

Approximately one-third of meniscal tears can be treated with conservative therapy consisting of exercises, bracing, and oral medications. The other two-thirds often require surgical intervention because of interference with activities of daily living or sports.

The present surgical approaches are meniscal excision or repair (meniscoresis). Arthroscopic excision removes a portion of the meniscus in the area of the tear. This decreases the area of contact and affects all the parameters

Table 7-1. Meniscal Tears: Incidence of Occurrence

Medial Meniscus
  posterior flap
  vertical longitudinal
  bucket handle
  radial

Lateral Meniscus
  radial
  vertical longitudinal
  bucket handle
  flap

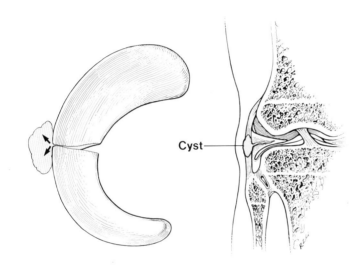

Cyst

Fig. 7-14. A cyst emanating from a meniscal tear.

reviewed in Chapter 2. The long term studies of arthroscopic excision have not yet been completed; however, the results appear to be satisfactory. Total meniscectomy in the past, however, has been associated with a slight increase in degenerative joint disease several years later.

Meniscal repair has even shorter follow-up. The perioperative complications are higher and the long term findings will have to be documented. The failure rate of repair is somewhere in the range of 10 to 50 percent depending upon the surgeon's experience, the age of the patient, the location of the tear, and the age of the tear. Increased experience enables one to become more proficient and perform the procedure with greater skill and better decision making. Younger patients seem to have a higher success rate of healing tears, probably because the tears in this age group are less complex and are not commonly degenerative. Tears that are chronic cause greater destruction to the blood supply and to the meniscus body.

The surgical approach to the meniscus should be tempered by any associated ligamentous injury and by the axial alignment of the knee. For example, the anterior cruciate deficient knee is not a good setting for meniscal repair because the repair will be subject to the abnormal anterolateral rotatory instability. Therefore, if repair is being considered, the knee must have adequate ligamentous stability.

A second consideration is the axial alignment. If the knee is in a varus position, medial meniscectomy may lead to an increase in this varus and may increase the very pain that the surgeon is trying to alleviate. Secondly, a medial meniscus repair (ill advised in the older population in general) may also be doomed to failure because of a pre-existing varus deformity with resultant increased stress on the side of the surgery.

SUGGESTED READINGS

Adams ME, McDevitt CA, Ho A, Muir H: Isolation and characterization of high-buoyant-density proteoglycans from semilunar menisci. J Bone Joint Surg [Am] 1986 Jan;68(1):55–64

Albertsson M, Gillquist J: Discoid lateral menisci: a report of 29 cases. Arthroscopy 1988;4(3):211–4

Appel H: Late results after meniscectomy in the knee joint. A clinical and roentgenologic follow-up investigation. Acta Orthop Scand Suppl 1970;133:Suppl 133:1+

**Arnoczky SP, Warren RF: The microvasculature of the meniscus and its response to injury. An experimental study in the dog. Am J Sports Med 1983 May–Jun;11(3):131–41

Barrie HJ: The pathogenesis and significance of menisceal cysts. J Bone Joint Surg [Br] 1979 May;61-B(2):184–9

Burr DB, Radin EL: Meniscal function and the importance of meniscal regeneration in preventing late medical compartment osteoarthrosis. Clin Orthop 1982 Nov–Dec;(171):121–6

*Cameron HU, Macnab I: The structure of the meniscus of the human knee joint. Clin Orthop 1972;89:215–9

Casscells SW: The torn meniscus, the torn anterior cruciate ligament, and their relationship to degenerative joint disease. Arthroscopy 1985;1(1):28–32

Day B, Mackenzie WG, Shim SS, Leung G: The vascular and nerve supply of the human meniscus. Arthroscopy 1985;1(1):58–62

*DeHaven KE: Rationale for meniscus repair or excision. Clin Sports Med 1985 Apr;4(2):267–73

Dickason JM, Del Pizzo W, Blazina ME et al: A series of ten discoid medial menisci. Clin Orthop 1982 Aug;(168):75–9

Fowler PJ, Lubliner JA: The predictive value of five clinical signs in the evaluation of meniscal pathology. Arthroscopy 1989;5(3):184–6

Gallo GA, Bryan RS: Cysts of the semilunar cartilages of the knee. Am J Surg 1968 Jul;116(1):65–8

Gronblad M, Korkala O, Liesi P, Karaharju E: Innervation of synovial membrane and meniscus. Acta Orthop Scand 1985 Dec;56(6):484–6

Henning CE, Lynch MA: Current concepts of meniscal function and pathology. Clin Sports Med 1985 Apr;4(2):259–65

Hernandex FJ: Cysts of the semilunar cartilage of the knee. A light and electron microscopic study. Acta Orthop Scand 1976 Aug;47(4):436–40

Johnson RG, Simmons EH: Discoid medical meniscus. Clin Orthop 1982 Jul;(167):176–9

Krause WR, Pope MH, Johnson RJ, Wilder DG: Mechanical changes in the knee after meniscectomy. J Bone Joint Surg [Am] 1976 Jul;58(5):599–604

Levy IM, Torzilli PA, Gould JD, Warren RF: The effect of lateral meniscectomy on motion of the knee. J Bone Joint Surg [Am] 1989 Mar;71(3):401–6

Levy IM, Torzilli PA, Warren RF: The effect of medial meniscectomy on anterior-posterior motion of the knee. J Bone Joint Surg [Am] 1982 Jul;64(6):883–8

Manzione M, Pizzutillo PD, Peoples AB, Schweizer PA: Meniscectomy in children: a long-term follow-up study. Am J Sports Med 1983 May–Jun;11(3):111–5

Mariani PP, Puddu G: Meniscal ossicle. A case report. Am J Sports Med 1981 Nov–Dec;9(6):392–3

*Noble J: Lesions of the menisci. Autopsy incidence in adults less than fifty-five years old. J Bone Joint Surg [Am] 1977 Jun;59(4):480–3

Noble J, Hamblen DL: The pathology of the degenerate meniscus lesion. J Bone Joint Surg [Br] 1975 May;57(2):180–6

Northmore-Ball MD, Dandy DJ: Long-term results of arthroscopic partial menisectomy. Clin Orthop 1982 Jul;(167):34–42

Oretorp N, Alm A, Ekstrom H, Gillquist J: Immediate effects of meniscectomy on the knee joint. The effects of tensile load on knee joint ligaments in dogs. Acta Orthop Scand 1978 Aug;49(4):407–14

Pettrone FA: Meniscectomy: arthrotomy versus arthroscopy. Am J Sports Med 1982 Nov–Dec;10(6):355–9

Radin EL, Bryan RS: The effect of weight-bearing on regrowth of the medial meniscus after meniscectomy. J Trauma 1970 Feb;10(2):169–75

Radin EL, de Lamotte F, Maquet P: Role of the menisci in the distribution of stress in the knee. Clin Orthop 1984 May;(185):290–4

Renstrom P, Johnson RJ: Anatomy and biomechanics of the menisci. Clin Sports Med 1990 Jul;9(3):523–38

Shoemaker SC, Markolf KL: The role of the meniscus in the anterior-posterior stability of the loaded anterior cruciate-deficient knee. Effects of partial versus total excision. J Bone Joint Surg [Am] 1986 Jan;68(1):71–9

Stener B: Unusual ganglion cysts in the neighbourhood of the knee joint. A report of six cases—three with involvement of the peroneal nerve. Acta Orthop Scand 1969;40(3):392–401

Symeonides PP, Ioannides G: Ossicles in the knee menisci. Report of three cases. J Bone Joint Surg [Am] 1972 Sep;54(6):1288–92

Tudisco C, Conteduca F, Puddu G: Synovial hemangioma of the meniscal wall simulating a meniscal cyst. A case report. Am J Sports Med 1988 Mar–Apr;16(2):191–2

Vahvanen V, Aalto K: Meniscectomy in children. Acta Orthop Scand 1979 Dec;50(6 Pt 2):791–5

**Walker PS, Erkman MJ: The role of the menisci in force transmission across the knee. Clin Orthop 1975;(109):184–92

** Source reference
* Reference of major interest

Fractures   **8**

This chapter will discuss pediatric and adult fractures about the knee. Growth plate injuries require a different approach from that of the adult fractures and must be considered separately.

Fracture treatment is also affected by the possibility of an associated compounding wound. Compound injuries are classified into three main groups according to the extent of displacement and associated soft tissue injury. Type I fractures have minimal wounds and have a good prognosis. Type III fractures have significant soft tissue injury and compromise of the vessels or nerves.

The description of any fracture should include the bone involved, location in the bone, relationship to any existing epiphysis or joint surface, displacement, angulation, and any compounding wounds.

PEDIATRIC FRACTURES

Each fracture should be classified as to its location with respect to the open epiphysis. Thus, the diaphysis, metaphysis, and epiphysis must be identified. If the fracture is in the metaphysis or diaphysis and does not violate the growth plate, then the prognosis is better and one can often accept slight displacements without a compromised result.

If the fracture crosses the growth plate, one must be more precise so that the plate is anatomically reduced. The Salter-Harris classification from I to V has been used to indicate the prognosis for each type of fracture involving the epiphysis (Fig. 8-1). Salter I fractures open the growth plate. Salter II fractures have an extension into the metaphysis. This fragment is referred to as the Thurston-Holland fragment. Salter III fractures extend from the growth plate into the epiphysis. Salter IV fractures extend across both the epiphysis and the metaphysis. Salter V fractures crush the growth plate. Type I fractures have the best prognosis for healing without growth disturbance and Type V have the worst prognosis.

Along with the description of the growth plate injury, the degree of displacement must also be noted. The undisplaced fracture is treated with immobilization and observation. The displaced fracture indicates greater force and injury. A reduction must be accomplished, and the prognosis is not as good.

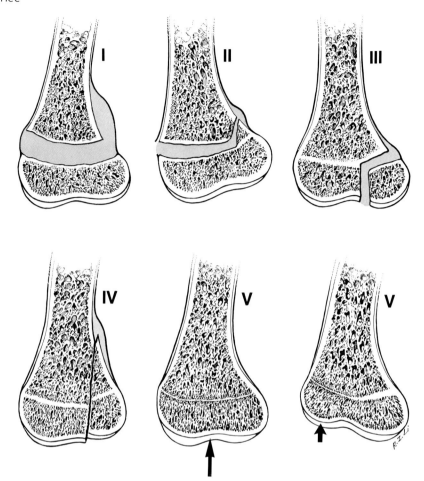

Fig. 8-1. The Salter-Harris classification includes five fracture patterns about the growth plate with the prognosis worsening from type I to type V.

Femoral Fractures

Supracondylar femoral fractures (above the epiphysis) can be treated with traction and/or casts if displacement is minimal. These injuries do not commonly require open reduction and heal well. On the anteroposterior (AP) or lateral roentgenogram one can accept displacement of one-half of the shaft diameter. On the lateral roentgenogram one can accept flexion or extension of the distal fragment of up to 10 degrees, and on the AP one can accept 5 degrees of medial or lateral angulation (Fig. 8-2). Deviations outside these guidelines require reduction of the fracture.

The supracondylar and condylar fractures that violate the growth plate are most commonly Salter I, II, and III fractures; they require an anatomic reduction. Occasionally, this can be accomplished with closed techniques; however, it is often necessary to perform an open reduction and hold the fragments with some form of pin or screw fixation. The plates and intramedullary devices used for adult fractures are not used for children so as to minimize injury to the growth plate. If at all possible, the surgeon tries not to place any fixation devices across the growth plate itself.

The displaced Salter I fracture can usually be reduced without internal fixation.

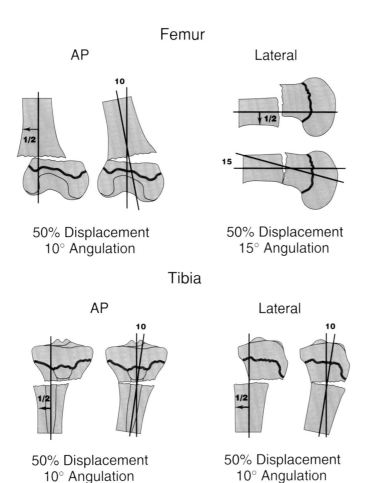

Fig. 8-2. Metaphyseal reduction criteria for children.

The displaced Salter II fracture of the distal femur can be a very deceptive injury. Its prognosis is not as good as the classification would imply because of possible rotation of the fragments that is not entirely clear on the standard films; therefore, the fracture should be reduced anatomically for the best possible result. It is often possible to pin the Thurston-Holland fragment to the remaining metaphysis and hold the reduction without violating the growth plate.

The displaced Salter III usually requires surgical intervention with fixation across the distal condyles without crossing the growth plate.

The displaced Salter IV fractures are rarely seen in the distal femur but usually require internal fixation. The Salter V injury crushes the growth plate but seldom displaces very much (Fig. 8-1).

Tibial Fractures

The tibial metaphyseal fractures that do not violate the growth plate can be treated similarly to the femoral type fractures discussed above. They should be reduced as adequately as possible and placed in traction or casts as

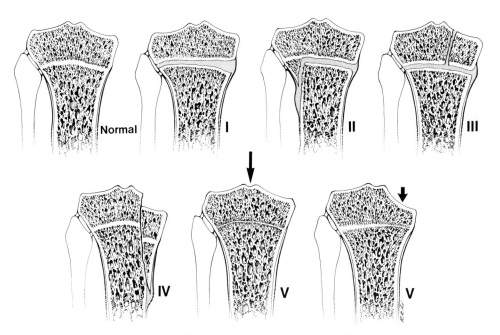

Fig. 8-3. Salter fractures of the proximal tibia.

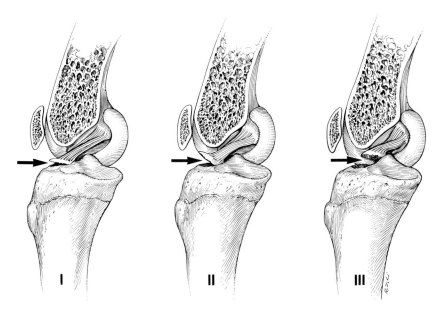

Fig. 8-4. There are three fractures of the tibial eminence. Type I and II are usually reduced with closed techniques. Type III may occasionally require open reduction.

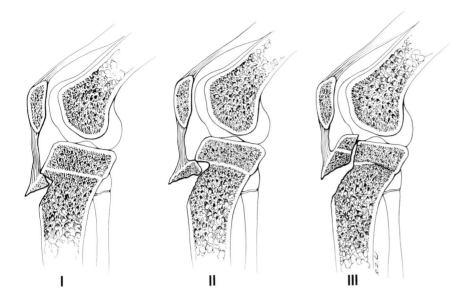

I   II   III

Fig. 8-5. There are three tibial tubercle fractures. Type I and II may reduce with extension of the knee. Type III is a Salter III injury and often requires open reduction.

deemed appropriate. Displacement of the shaft fragment by one-half of the entire width on the AP or lateral view, angulation of up to 5 degrees on the AP view, and angulation of up to 10 degrees on the lateral view are acceptable parameters (Fig. 8-2). Surgery is not commonly necessary.

The epiphyseal injuries to the proximal tibia are usually Salter I and II. The displaced Salter I is most often reduced closed. The displaced Salter II is usually reduced closed and does not have the added risks seen in the femoral Salter II. The displaced Salter III and IV fractures are rarely seen on the tibial side and usually require open reduction. The Salter V is also rare and usually is not displaced but has the worst prognosis (Fig. 8-3).

Along with the epiphyseal injuries, the proximal tibia is also subject to eminence fractures. These fractures are most common in the skeletally immature and are seldom seen in the adult population, in whom injury to the anterior cruciate is more common.

There are three types of eminence fractures: The first type does not involve displacement and can be treated with immobilization; the second type is lifted up from the bed with the opening anterior and usually is reduced with extension of the knee; the third type displaces the entire eminence from the plateau surface and becomes parallel to the surface. The latter fracture can sometimes be closed reduced but may often require open reduction and internal fixation (Fig. 8-4).

There are also three avulsion fractures of the tibial tubercle. The Type I fracture occurs just at the insertion of the patellar ligament. Type II fractures occur at the junction of the apophyseal area with the transverse growth plate. Type III fractures cross the epiphysis into the joint surface because the posterior tibial physis is closed. The Type I and II injuries are often reduced with full extension of the knee. The Type III is a Salter III fracture and must be reduced anatomically; this often necessitates open reduction (Fig. 8-5).

Fibular Fractures

Proximal fibular fractures can present with the same Salter patterns but are less worrisome because the fibula does not effect the growth of the lower leg as much as the tibia does. If the tibia is appropriately reduced, the fibular fracture usually follows suite and also reduces.

Patella fragmentations

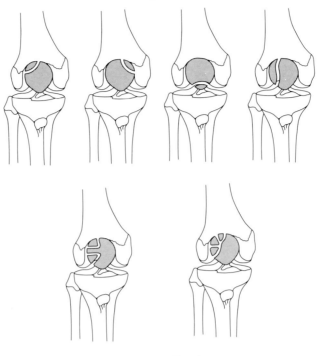

Patella duplications

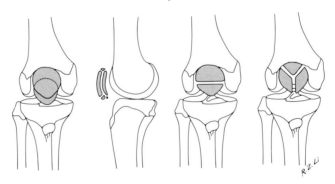

Fig. 8-6. The patellar dysplasias and duplications may occasionally be confused with an acute fracture.

Patellar Fractures

Patellar fractures are uncommon in the youth. When roentgenographic changes are noted, one must be careful not to confuse dysplasias with true fractures (Fig. 8-6). The fracture patterns seen in the adult (Fig. 8-12) can occur but are extremely unusual and seldom involve disruption of the extensor mechanism.

ADULT FRACTURES

Femoral Fractures

The adult distal femur is subject to supracondylar, intercondylar, condylar, and osteochondral fracture. Neer, Shelton, and Grantham classified the supra- and intracondylar fractures with respect to the intercondylar component and the femoral shaft displacement (Fig. 8-7). The Type I fracture is T shaped, extends into the joint between the condyles, but involves minimal displacement. The Type IIA is also a T, but the femoral shaft is displaced laterally. The Type IIB is also a T, but the femoral shaft is displaced medially. The Type III is a supracondylar fracture without intercondylar extension but with metaphyseal comminution. All of these fractures are initially reduced with traction techniques to see if adequate reduction is possible. The criteria are similar to those described above for the immature femur but are slightly more stringent because of the minimal remodelling that is possible. Displacement of the femoral shaft medially or laterally of 50 percent of the shaft width is acceptable. The varus or valgus angulation must be below 5 degrees and the flexion/extension angulation below 10 degrees. Displacement of the intercondylar component must be less than two mm (Fig. 8-8). If these parameters cannot be satisfied, then open reduction becomes necessary.

Condylar fractures of the femur are less common. They occur in the sagittal and coronal planes (Fig. 8-9). The sagittal fractures involve one or both condyles without a significant metaphyseal extension. The coronal fracture usually involves the posterior portion of the condyle. Because of the intra-articular nature of these fractures, they require accurate reductions within 1 or 2 mm, often necessitating operative intervention.

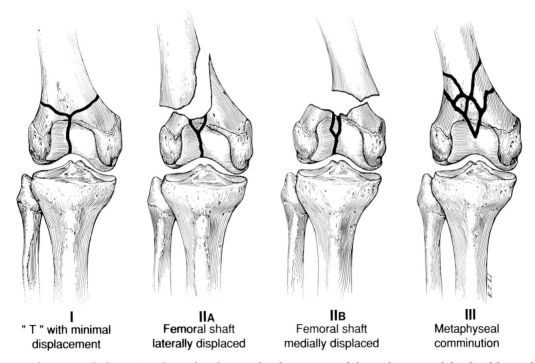

I	IIA	IIB	III
" T " with minimal displacement	Femoral shaft laterally displaced	Femoral shaft medially displaced	Metaphyseal comminution

Fig. 8-7. The Neer, Shelton, Grantham classification for the supracondylar and intercondylar distal femur fracture.

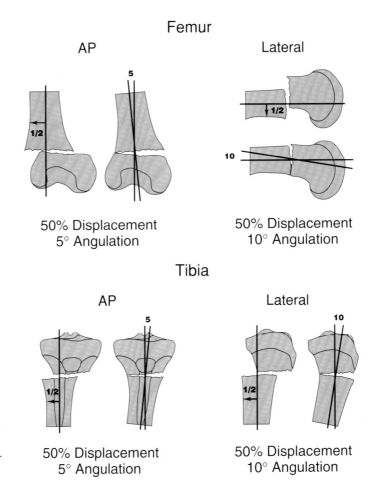

Femur

AP   Lateral

50% Displacement   50% Displacement
5° Angulation   10° Angulation

Tibia

AP   Lateral

Fig. 8-8. Metaphyseal reduction criteria for adults.

50% Displacement   50% Displacement
5° Angulation   10° Angulation

Fig. 8-9. Condylar fractures of the femur occur in the sagittal and coronal planes.

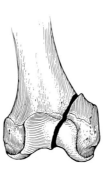

Medial condyle
fracture

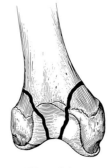

Bicondylar
fracture

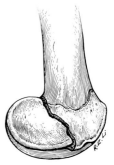

Posterior condyle
fracture

Osteochondral fractures can occur in almost any location along the femoral articular surface, depending upon the myriad of different mechanisms of injury. A common fracture involves the lateral aspect of the lateral femoral condyle in association with patellar dislocation (Fig. 8-10A). They may also be seen when a preexisting surface abnormality (such as osteochondritis dissecans of the lateral wall of the medial femoral condyle) is subjected to new

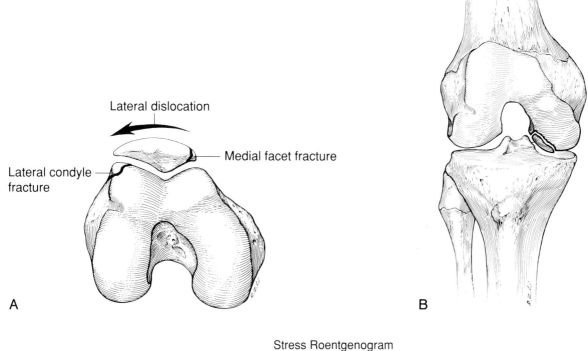

A

B

Stress Roentgenogram

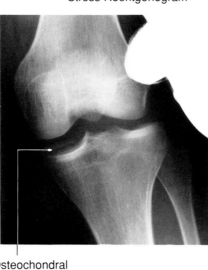

C

Fig. 8-10. (A) Osteochondral fracture of the lateral femoral condyle in association with patellar dislocation. (B) Osteochondral fracture of a preexisting osteochondritis dissecans of the lateral wall of the medial femoral condyle. (C) Osteochondral fracture of the posterior medial aspect of the tibial plateau rim in association with a combined medial collateral, anterior, and posterior cruciate ligament disruption without knee dislocation.

trauma and a fragment is released (Fig. 8-10B). Severe trauma to the joint (as in knee dislocation) may lead to osteochondral lesions in unpredictable locations (Fig. 8-10C). The fractures are often difficult to identify and involve the hyaline cartilage along with some of the underlying subchondral bone. If the bone fragment is extremely small, there may be only a fleck of calcification on the roentgenogram to indicate the area of fracture. Thus, one's index of suspicion must be high and associated injuries must also be considered. The treatment is most often excision of the fragment, unless it includes a significant portion of the weight-bearing surface. If the area is important, then attempts must be made to secure the fragment back into its anatomic bed. This is often mechanically difficult and fraught with complications.

Tibial Fractures

Fractures of the proximal tibia involve the tibial articular surface, the eminences (less common in adults), and the metaphysis. Plateau fractures can be classified as compressed, split, compressed and split, condylar, and comminuted. Mason Hohl's classification is the most commonly used description (Fig. 8-11).

The major difficulty with this group of fractures is the determination of acceptable displacement. The literature indicates limits from 4 to 14 mm for the depression or the split. Tomograms and CT scans are helpful, but often the decision for or against open reduction is a subjective one affected by the age of the patient, level of activity, overall medical health, and the roentgenographic presentation.

Eminence fractures are uncommon in adults and can be treated with the same guidelines (the three types and the degree of displacement) as in the immature population. In the adult knee it appears that the anterior cruciate ligament disrupts before the bone fractures.

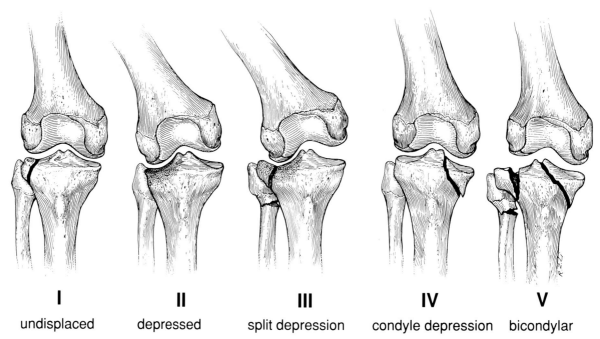

I	II	III	IV	V
undisplaced	depressed	split depression	condyle depression	bicondylar

Fig. 8-11. Fractures of the tibial plateau are classified according to depression, split, and the area of condylar involvement. (Modified from Hohl M: Tibial condylar fractures. J Bone Joint Surg [Am] 1967;49:1455–1467, with permission.)

Metaphyseal fractures can usually be treated with an appropriate closed reduction and immobilization. The reduction must be subjected to limits of 50 percent shaft displacement medial to lateral or anterior to posterior. Varus or valgus angulation cannot exceed 5 degrees. Flexion or extension angulation cannot exceed 10 degrees (Fig. 8-8). If these criteria cannot be satisfied, then open reduction must be considered.

Patellar Fractures

Fractures of the patella can be divided into the undisplaced, transverse, distal pole, proximal pole, comminuted, and vertical (Fig. 8-12). The keys to treatment are the extensor mechanism and the degree of displacement. The transverse, distal, or proximal pole fractures may occasionally result in loss of the extensor mechanism because of extension of the fracture injury into the medial and lateral retinaculum. If this is the case, then surgical intervention becomes necessary both to restore articular congruity and the extensor integrity.

If any of the fractures results in displacement of more than 2 mm, surgery is usually necessary to maintain articular congruity. This is usually accomplished with a circular wire around the patella or interfragmentary screws.

The patellar dysplasias discussed in Chapter 10 must not be confused with acute fractures (Fig. 8-6). However, it is possible that injury to a preexisting dysplastic area, such as a secondary ossification center or osteochondritis dissecans, can lead to displacement that was not present before.

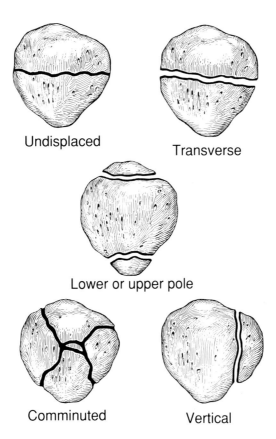

Undisplaced   Transverse

Lower or upper pole

Comminuted   Vertical

Fig. 8-12. Fractures of the patella.

DISLOCATIONS

Patellar Dislocation

Patellar dislocations are most commonly lateral and occur in the first 30 degrees from full extension. They can be associated with fracture of either the lateral femoral condyle or the medial patellar facet. Reduction is accomplished with manual pressure in full extension. If there is a displaced fragment, operative intervention may be necessary; otherwise, the initial dislocation is treated with immobilization and range of motion after 4 to 6 weeks. The recurrence rate is 30 percent in the younger age group (less than 20 years old) and decreases to 5 percent in the age group over forty years old.

Medial dislocations are rare and are most commonly iatrogenic (as in association with extensor mechanism realignment procedures in which the medial reefing is overdone). Intra-articular dislocations have also been described in which the patella turns horizontally into the joint between the femoral condyles and the tibial plateau surface. Both of these dislocations are difficult to diagnose and often require operative intervention.

Femorotibial Dislocation

Dislocation of the knee joint itself is a severe but fortunately uncommon injury. The dislocation can occur in any of the four directions about the knee and may be associated with a fracture. If there is no associated fracture, then at least three of the four major ligaments are disrupted in order for the displacement to occur. Injury to the popliteal artery or the major nerves (peroneal before the tibial) occurs in up to 50 percent of the cases reported in the literature. The extensor mechanism is sometimes injured, with the disruption leading to patellar dislocation or rupture of the patellar ligament insertion into the tibial tubercle.

Anterior dislocation has the highest association with injury to the popliteal artery. This may lead to complete transection of the vessel or to intimal wall tear. The latter insult can be difficult to diagnose without an arteriogram because the distal pulses can be completely intact. Thus, one's index of suspicion should be high and the vascular anatomy clearly delineated.

Posterolateral dislocation has the highest association with injury to the peroneal and tibial nerves. Usually the nerve is stretched, but on occasion the root may be completely disrupted.

These injuries are primarily treated with surgical repairs to allow early motion and avoid severe loss of range of motion associated with cast immobilization. The collateral ligaments with the posteromedial and posterolateral capsular structures should be the primary surgical focus. The cruciate ligaments may or may not be repairable and are not as important for the final result as are the collaterals. The repairs should be completed with enough care so that motion can be instituted as soon as possible. Compartment syndromes are not uncommon, either before or after the surgery, and they should always be suspected. If there are associated fractures, they should be approached according to the outline established above, with the knowledge that fixation must be adequate to allow early motion.

Tibiofibular Dislocation

Dislocation of the tibiofibular joint as an isolated event is even more uncommon than knee joint dislocation. The displacement can occur in all four directions but is usually seen either anteriorly or posteriorly. Reduction can be accomplished manually and is usually stable with a very low incidence of recurrence (10 percent). The anterior injury is often associated with peroneal nerve compromise secondary to stretch of the nerve.

SUGGESTED READINGS

**Aichroth P: Osteochondritis dissecans of the knee. J Bone Joint Surg [Br] 1971;53:440–7

*Bostrom A: Fracture of the patella. A study of 422 patellar fractures. Acta Orthop Scand Suppl 1972;143:1–80

Bowers KD Jr: Patellar tendon avulsion as a complication of Osgood-Schlatter's disease. Am J Sports Med 1981 Nov–Dec;9(6):356–9

Bowes DN, Hohl M: Tibial condylar fractures. Evaluation of treatment and outcome. Clin Orthop 1982 Nov–Dec;(171):104–8

Campbell CJ, Ranawat CS: Osteochondritis dissecans: the question of etiology. J Trauma 1966 Mar;6(2):201–21

Crawford AH: Fractures about the knee in children. Orthop Clin North Am 1976 Jul;7(3):639–56

Delamarter RB, Hohl M, Hopp E Jr: Ligament injuries associated with tibial plateau fractures. Clin Orthop 1990 Jan;(250):226–33

Egund N, Kolmert L: Deformities, gonarthrosis and function after distal femoral fractures. Acta Orthop Scand 1982 Dec;53(6):963–74

Goldman AB, Pavlov H, Rubenstein D: The Segond fracture of the proximal tibia: a small avulsion that reflects major ligamentous damage. AJR Am J Roentgenol 1988 Dec;151(6):1163–7

Healy WL, Brooker AF Jr: Distal femoral fractures. Comparison of open and closed methods of treatment. Clin Orthop 1983 Apr;(174):166–71

**Hohl M: Tibial condylar fractures. J Bone Joint Surg [Am] 1967;49:1455–1467

Jerosch JG, Castro WH, Jantea C: Stress fracture of the patella. Am J Sports Med 1989 Jul–Aug;17(4):579–80

**Kennedy JC: Complete dislocation of the knee joint. J Bone Joint Surg [Am] 1963;45:889–904

Kennedy JC, Grainger RW, McGraw RW: Osteochondral fractures of the femoral condyles. J Bone Joint Surg [Br] 1966 Aug;48(3):436–40

Kolmert L, Wulff K: Epidemiology and treatment of distal femoral fractures in adults. Acta Orthop Scand 1982 Dec;53(6):957–62

Letts M, Vincent N, Gouw G: The "floating knee" in children. J Bone Joint Surg [Br] 1986 May;68(3):442–6

Lewis SL, Pozo JL, Muirhead-Allwood WF: Coronal fractures of the lateral femoral condyle. J Bone Joint Surg [Br] 1989 Jan;71(1):118–20

*Lombardo SJ, Harvey JP Jr: Fractures of the distal femoral epiphyses. Factors influencing prognosis: a review of thirty-four cases. J Bone Joint Surg [Am] 1977 Sep;59(6):742–51

*Meyers MH, Moore TM, Harvey JP Jr: Traumatic dislocation of the knee joint. J Bone Joint Surg [Am] 1975 Apr;57(3):430–3

Milgram JW, Rogers LF, Miller JW: Osteochondral fractures: mechanisms of injury and fate of fragments. AJR Am J Roentgenol 1978 Apr;130(4):651–8

Mooney V: Fractures of the distal femur. Instr Course Lect 1987;36:427

*Moore TM: Fracture—dislocation of the knee. Clin Orthop 1981 May;(156):128–40

**Neer CS 2d, Grantham SA, Shelton ML: Supracondylar fracture of the adult femur. A study of one hundred and ten cases. J Bone Joint Surg [Am] 1967 Jun;49(4):591–613

O'Donoghue DH: Chondral and osteochondral fractures. J Trauma 1966 Jul;6(4):469–81

**Ogden JA: Subluxation and dislocation of the proximal tibiofibular joint. J Bone Joint Surg [Am] 1974 Jan;56(1):145–154

Odgen JA, Tross RB, Murphy MJ: Fractures of the tibial tuberosity in adolescents. J Bone Joint Surg [Am] 1980;62:205–215

** Source reference
* Reference of major interest

Olerud S: Operative treatment of supracondylar–condylar fractures of the femur. Technique and results in fifteen cases. J Bone Joint Surg [Am] 1972 Jul;54(5):1015–32

*Rasmussen PS: Tibial condylar fractures: Impairment of knee joint stability as an indication for surgical treatment. J Bone Joint Surg [Am] 1973;55:1331–1350

Riggins RS, Garrick JG, Lipscomb PR: Supracondylar fractures of the femur. A survey of treatment. Clin Orthop 1972 Jan–Feb;82:32–6

Roberts JM: Operative treatment of fractures about the knee. Orthop Clin North Am 1990 Apr;21(2):365–79

Rorabeck CH, Bobechko WP: Acute dislocation of the patella with osteochondral fracture: a review of eighteen cases. J Bone Joint Surg [Br] 1976 May;58(2):237–40

Rosenthal RK, Levine DB: Fragmentation of the distal pole of the patella in spastic cerebral palsy. J Bone Joint Surg [Am] 1977 Oct;59(7):934–9

*Schatzker J, McBroom R, Bruce D: The tibial plateau fracture. The Toronto experience 1968–1975. Clin Orthop 1979 Jan–Feb;(138):94–104

Scheller S, Martenson L: Traumatic dislocation of the patella. A radiographic investigation. Acta Radiol Suppl (Stockh) 1974;336:1–160

Seinsheimer F 3d: Fractures of the distal femur. Clin Orthop 1980 Nov–Dec;(153):169–79

Shields L, Mital M, Cave EF: Complete dislocation of the knee: experience at the Massachusetts General Hospital. J Trauma 1969 Mar;9(3):192–215

Waldrop JI, Macey TI, Trettin JC et al: Fractures of the posterolateral tibial plateau. Am J Sports Med 1988 Sep–Oct;16(5):492–8

Zimmerman AJ: Intra-articular fractures of the distal femur. Orthop Clin North Am 1979 Jan;10(1):75–80

Arthritis
Diagnosis and Treatment

9

Arthritis of the knee can be divided into five major categories: osteoarthritis, inflammatory arthritis, metabolic arthritis, infectious arthritis, and the neuropathic joint.

The initial evaluation of the patient should include a complete history. The most common presenting complaint is pain. Instability or mechanical locking and, occasionally, painless swelling may also be included in the symptom complex. The nature of the pain should be characterized in terms of its location within the knee, type of onset (sudden or gradual), duration, relationship to weight-bearing and/or injury, and presence at rest or at night while sleeping. The examiner should also establish if the knee is the only area involved or if multiple joints are concerned.

PHYSICAL EXAMINATION

The examination should include all of the parameters outlined in Chapter 3. On evaluation of the gait and stance one should note other joint involvement and the use of any supportive devices (crutches, cane, wheelchair). The range of motion, any clinical deformity (varus, valgus, or flexion), evidence of effusion, joint line crepitation, and specific areas of tenderness should all be noted.

LABORATORY TESTS

The laboratory evaluation should include the complete blood count, an erythrocyte sedimentation rate, rheumatoid factor, antinuclear antibody test, human leucocyte antigen (HLA) B27, lyme titer, electrolytes, serum calcium, phosphorous, alkaline phosphatase, uric acid, blood sugar, blood urea nitrogen (BUN), creatinine, serum glutamic oxaloacetic transaminase (SGOT), lactic dehydrogenase (LDH), and globulin level.

The urinalysis should include the report of the protein, cell count, and the presence or absence of stones.

Finally, the knee joint may need to be aspirated for diagnostic purposes. The authors do not feel that the knee should be drained routinely and do not recommend intra-articular injections of steroids because of the possibility of introducing infection or of causing injury to the lamina splendens covering of the hyaline cartilage. The most common reason to obtain fluid should be to confirm the possibility of infection. Most other arthritic diagnoses can be

Table 9-1. Synovial Fluid Analysis

Parameter Evaluated	Normal Knee	Type of Arthritis		
		Osteoarthritis	Inflammatory Arthritis	Septic Arthritis
Volume	<4cc	often >4cc	often >4cc	often >4cc
Clarity	transparent	transparent	translucent	opaque
Color	clear	yellow	yellow to green	yellow to green
Viscosity	high	high	low	variable
Mucin Clot	good	good	fair	poor
Spontaneous Clot	no	often	often	often
WBC/mm3	<200	200–2,000	2,000–75,000	>100,000
Polymorphonuclear leucocytes	<25%	<25%	>70%	>90%
Glucose	= FBS	= FBS	slightly <FBS	<FBS
Protein (GM%)	<2.5	<2.5	>2.5	>2.5
Culture	negative	negative	negative	positive
Example Diseases		Avascular Necrosis Degenerative Joint Disease Ochronosis Osteochondritis Dissecans Paget's Sickle Cell Trauma Tumors	Ankylosing Spondylitis Gout Lyme Pseudogout Psoriatic Reiter's Rheumatic Fever Rheumatoid Sarcoidosis	Bacterial Infection Tuberculosis

made without knee joint fluid. Table 9-1 outlines the laboratory analysis of the fluid that may be obtained.

ROENTGENOGRAPHIC STUDIES

The plain roentgenograms form one of the primary tests for underlying arthritis. All of the conditions include loss of the normal joint space in one or more areas of the knee. The bone may be sclerotic or osteoporotic and may include osteophyte formation or subchondral cysts. The cysts may be central or peripheral. The soft tissue is often involved with either a symmetric or asymmetric appearance. During the early phases of arthritis of the knee, the evolving changes are usually clear and help in the diagnostic evaluation. As the involvement of the joint progresses, the joint destruction becomes more diffuse and the roentgenographic changes all become similar in their appearance. Table 9-2 summarizes the changes seen on x-ray. While these criteria are not diagnostic by themselves, combined with the history, physical examination, and laboratory tests, they should point to a very specific disease entity.

CLINICAL PRESENTATIONS

Osteoarthritis

Osteoarthritis of the knee is most commonly idiopathic; however, several other entities (such as trauma, avascular necrosis, pigmented villonodular

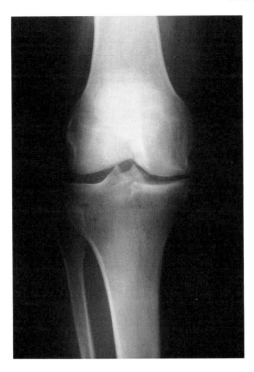

Fig. 9-1. Roentgenogram illustrating osteoarthritis with joint space narrowing, sclerosis, and osteophytes.

synovitis, and blood dyscrasias with recurrent hemarthroses and subsequent joint injury) can lead to a similar roentgenographic picture.

Idiopathic osteoarthritis presents in the older population with multiple joint involvement of varying intensities. Varus or neutral alignment of the knee is most common, with some loss of the extremes of extension and flexion. Crepitation is palpable along the joint lines, and an effusion is often present. The laboratory data is within normal limits. The synovial fluid will have a high viscosity, with good mucin clot, a mild leukocytosis (less than 2,000 WBC/mm3) with predominantly mononuclear cells, a normal sugar and a low protein level. The roentgenograms demonstrate joint space narrowing (often on just the medial or just the lateral side), sclerosis, osteophytes, and central subchondral cysts (Figure 9-1).

Inflammatory Arthritis

This category includes psoriatic arthritis, Reiter's syndrome, ankylosing spondylitis, sarcoidosis, rheumatic fever, gout, and pseudogout.

Rheumatoid arthritis is the major entity in inflammatory arthritis of the knee. There are two groups of patients: the juvenile and the adult. Both present with diffuse pain in the knee joint and morning stiffness. At the onset, the knee may be the only area of involvement, but as the disease progresses many other joints become affected. The distribution of the joint involvement is often diagnostic. Examination of the hand may be especially helpful because of the specific involvement of the metacarpalphalangeal and proximal interphalangeal joints with almost complete sparing of the distal interphalangeal joints.

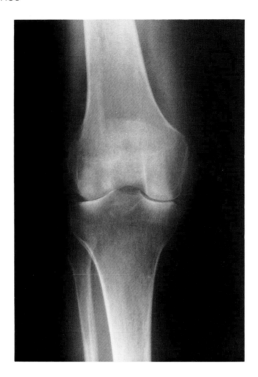

Fig. 9-2. Roentgenogram illustrating rheumatoid arthritis with diffuse narrowing and osteoporosis.

The physical examination of the knee reveals a diffuse symmetric soft tissue swelling with a boggy synovium. The knee often has a flexion contracture while varus and valgus deformities are less common. All areas of the knee are tender to palpation. Crepitation may be present along the joint lines but is not as common as in the osteoarthritic knee.

Laboratory tests may indicate a positive rheumatoid factor with a moderate elevation of the sedimentation rate and the peripheral white count. The synovial fluid will show low viscosity, fair to poor mucin clot, leukocytosis (2,000 to 75,000 WBC/mm3) with 70 percent polymorphonuclear leukocytes, slightly lower sugar level, and elevation of the protein level. A positive rheumatoid factor test for the synovial fluid is diagnostic for the disease entity. The synovial biopsy may show rheumatoid nodules. The roentgenograms reveal diffuse joint space narrowing, with osteoporosis, peripheral or marginal erosions, and symmetric soft tissue swelling. There is no sclerosis or osteophyte formation (Fig. 9-2).

Metabolic Arthritis

Metabolic arthritis of the knee can have many causes, such as *gout, pseudogout, chondrocalcinosis, ochronosis,* and *Paget's* disease. Patients present with symptoms similar to those of the osteoarthritic knee, with pain and swelling that increase with activity and weight-bearing. The physical examination will reveal the crepitation along the joint lines, some loss of range of motion, flexion contractures, occasional varus or valgus deformity, and asymmetric swelling with some evidence of lobulation of the underlying synovium.

Laboratory tests will be positive for the specific arthritic entity (such as an elevation of the serum uric acid in gout). The synovial fluid in Paget's disease

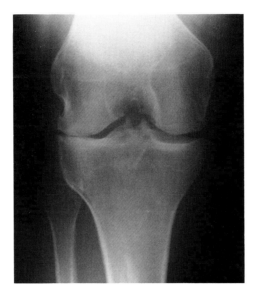

Fig. 9-3. Roentgenogram illustrating gout with joint space narrowing and sclerosis.

and ochronosis will be very similar to that of the osteoarthritic knee, with high viscosity, good mucin clot, low cell count (<2,000 WBC/mm3) with mononuclear cells predominating, normal sugar level, and low protein level.

Some of the metabolic diseases have an associated induced crystalline synovitis. *Gout* has strongly negative birefringent needle-shaped monosodium urate crystals. *Pseudogout* has positive birefringent rhomboid shaped calcium pyrophosphate crystals. Cholesterol and corticosteroid ester crystals (residuum from joint injections) may also be present and may confuse the picture. The steroid is seldom intracellular and there are enzymes that can be used to dissolve the pathogenic crystals, leaving the steroid and cholesterol behind to help in the diagnosis. The synovial fluid analysis in this group mimics that of inflammatory arthritis rather than osteoarthritis. The viscosity is low, the mucin clot fair, the WBC is 2,000 to 75,000 with 70 percent polymorphonuclear leucocytes, the glucose is slightly low, and the protein is elevated.

The roentgenograms will be similar to those of osteoarthritis with sclerosis, localized joint space narrowing, and some osteophytes. Early gout and pseudogout may look like inflammatory arthritis but convert to the osteoarthritis appearance as the disease advances. There may also be some marginal erosions with overhanging edges. The joint space is usually preserved in some areas of the knee. The menisci may reveal calcification. The soft tissue swelling is usually asymmetric (Fig. 9-3).

Infectious Arthritis

Infection in the knee is uncommon without an underlying cause. Once it has established itself in the joint, it is a difficult problem to eradicate. The patient

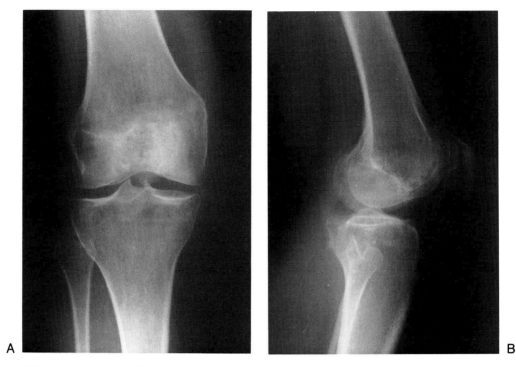

Fig. 9-4. (A) Anteroposterior and (B) lateral roentgenograms of the right knee with bacterial infection illustrating osteoporosis and symmetric swelling.

usually presents with a low-grade temperature and a swollen joint. The knee is held in slight flexion and weight-bearing is painful. Physical examination will document the effusion and tenderness in all areas of the knee. Inguinal adenopathy may also be present.

Laboratory blood tests will reveal a marked elevation of the erythrocyte sedimentation rate and mild elevation of the peripheral WBC count with the majority polymorphonuclear cells. The synovial fluid will have variable viscosity, opaque or cloudy appearance, poor mucin clot, a WBC count of greater than 100,000 cells/mm3 with the majority polymorphonuclear. The sugar level will be lower than the level in serum; the protein will be elevated; and the culture will usually be positive for the offending organism. The early roentgenograms may show nothing more than a suggestion of soft tissue swelling and osteoporosis (Fig. 9-4). As the infection progresses, the joint space will be destroyed and the soft tissue swelling will become more evident.

If the infection is limited to the joint space alone without invasion of the bone, the technetium and gallium scans will be negative, but there may be increased early flow. If the bone has been invaded, both the scans will be positive with more uptake evident on the gallium study.

The Neuropathic Joint

The neuropathic joint is the result of the loss of normal sensation (pain and/or proprioception) to the knee. This deficit leads to repetitious, undetected trauma. Charcot (in tabes dorsalis), Sokoloff (in syringomyelia), and Jordan (in

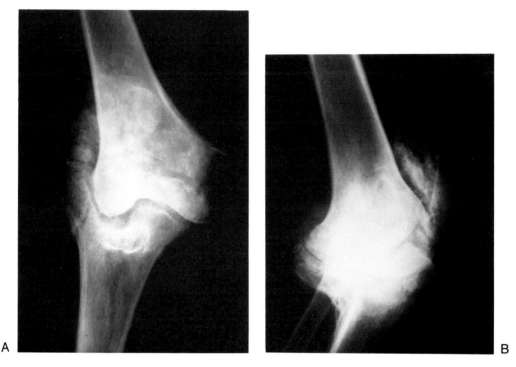

A   B

Fig. 9-5. (A) Anteroposterior and (B) lateral roentgenograms of a neuropathic joint illustrating joint space destruction with instability and periarticular debris.

diabetes mellitus) all described this entity. There are a myriad of causes including idiopathic, diabetic and alcoholic neuropathy, spinal cord tumors, and pernicious anemia. The patient usually presents in an atypical fashion because the joint is seldom painful. There may be swelling, deformity, or instability that brings the knee to the patient's attention.

The laboratory tests will support the diagnosis of the underlying disease (i.e., elevation of the blood sugar in diabetes, abnormal liver chemistries in alcoholic neuropathy). The synovial fluid analysis reveals findings similar to those of osteoarthritis with high viscosity, good mucin clot, low WBC count, normal sugar level, and low protein level.

The roentgenograms will show joint destruction with disorganization. There will be bone debris with calcification in the soft tissues, and the joint may show instability with translocation of the tibia beneath the femur in the standing position. The soft tissue swelling will be symmetrical, and osteoporosis is not as evident as in inflammatory or infectious arthritis (Fig. 9-5).

TREATMENT

Osteoarthritis, Inflammatory Arthritis, Metabolic Arthritis

The three primary arthritis categories are treated similarly. Once the diagnosis has been established, the treatment regimen begins with a simple *exercise* program for the knee, supportive *braces,* and oral *medications* that are either appropriate for the primary disease (e.g., indomethacin for gout or corticosteroids for rheumatoid arthritis) or anti-inflammatory drugs. The exercises

Table 9-2. Roentgenographic Changes
in Arthritis

Osteoarthritis
joint space narrowing (often localized)
subchondral sclerosis
osteophytes
subchondral cysts

Inflammatory Arthritis
diffuse joint space narrowing
absent subchondral sclerosis
absent osteophytes
subchondral cysts
osteoporosis
periarticular soft tissue swelling
(symmetric)

Metabolic Arthritis
localized joint space narrowing
marginal erosions
asymmetric soft tissue swelling
limited subchondral sclerosis
no osteoporosis
?chondrocalcinosis

Infectious Arthritis
joint space destroyed
joint effusion
symmetric soft tissue swelling
osteoporosis

Neuropathic Arthritis
joint space destroyed
periarticular debris
joint instability
joint effusion

keep proper tone in the surrounding musculature to support the joint. The braces help to give the patient subjective support while the knee is in the weight-bearing position. The primary medications control the underlying disease. The anti-inflammatory medications decrease the swelling and subsequent feeling of stiffness in the joint by decreasing the inflammatory response of the joint to the arthritis.

Supportive devices, such as a cane or a walker, help to transfer some of the weight to the upper extremities, thus unloading the joint during weight-bearing.

Failure of these conservative measures leads to surgical intervention. Surgery may be in the form of arthroscopy (for debridement), osteotomy (for alignment), or arthrotomy (for debridement, patellar alignment, or joint replacement). The choice of surgical intervention is influenced by the age of the patient, level of activity, type of arthritis, areas of involvement by symptom and by roentgenogram, the alignment of the knee, and the extent of the joint surface involvement.

Arthroscopy for arthritis is a limited procedure that removes degenerative changes in the menisci and smooths irregular surfaces. Attempts to encourage new hyaline cartilage development have been unsuccessful. Drilling of the subchondral bone does lead to fibrocartilage invasion, but the fibrocartilage does not have the properties of the normal cartilage and only provides fair relief of symptoms.

Arthroscopic synovectomy for inflammatory arthritis can be helpful if appropriately timed when the synovitis has progressed without significant articular surface destruction.

Realignment procedures correct abnormal tibiofemoral varus or valgus and lateral patellar tracking. The operations relieve pain in localized areas along the medial, lateral, and patellofemoral joint lines. Once again, these approaches cannot change the articular surface; they unload the involved area from increased pressure.

Arthrotomy of the knee for complete debridement (Magnuson or Pridie) is occasionally useful but has limited application.

Arthrotomy for *total joint arthroplasty* is very common and presently quite successful with the hope of 15 to 20 years of longevity for the implanted prostheses. The replacements require two different articulating surfaces (presently high density polyethylene on the tibial side and chrome-cobalt or a titanium alloy on the femoral side). They can be inserted with methylmethacrylate cement or with coated surfaces that encourage bone ingrowth without cement or with smooth surfaces that attempt to interlock with the bone (press fit).

Unicondylar replacements resurface the medial or lateral tibiofemoral joint, and some replacements resurface the patellofemoral joint; however, most arthroplasties resurface the entire knee joint. The collateral ligaments are preserved. The anterior cruciate ligament is sacrificed, and the posterior cruciate may be retained or removed depending upon the prosthetic design. All of the present prosthetic designs essentially resurface the knee, although some have more conformity between the femoral and tibial surfaces than others. Thus, the degree of "constraint" varies; however, very few prostheses incorporate a hinge articulation.

The indications for joint replacement are slightly different for the different categories of arthritis. The primary variable is the age at which replacement should be undertaken. In the rheumatoid population, surgery can be considered even in the early twenties if the other indications are present. The rheumatoid patient often has multiple joints involved, and the patient's life expectancy is shorter than that of the osteoarthritic patient.

Osteoarthritis and metabolic arthritis patients are usually in their mid to late fifties before replacement will be considered because these patients have a normal life expectancy and have only one or two major areas of involvement.

Most centers use a standard scoring system adapted either from the Hospital for Special Surgery or, more recently, from the Knee Society. The scores are derived from the evaluation of pain, the level of function, and the physical examination. Scores of 60 or lower usually support replacement. The roentgenograms should indicate total knee joint involvement, and the underlying diagnosis should be clearly established.

Infectious Arthritis

Knee joint infections require immediate attention. The diagnosis should be made with the support of the physical examination, the laboratory findings, the aspiration test results, and the roentgenographic presentation. Chapter 13 outlines the evaluation and treatment protocols.

Neuropathic Arthritis

It is most important that the correct diagnosis is made when evaluating neuropathic arthritis. The entity can often be confused with infection or with metabolic arthritis. Operative intervention is seldom indicated or successful in this entity. Debridement is unnecessary; replacement often leads to loosening because of the abnormal proprioception; and fusions have a high failure rate. Once the diagnosis is confirmed, it is best to support the knee with a walker, crutch, or cane along with some properly measured brace.

SUGGESTED READINGS

Aglietti P, Buzzi R: Idiopathic osteonecrosis of the knee. Ital J Orthop Traumatol 1984 Jun;10(2):217–26

Baumgaertner MR, Cannon WD Jr, Vittori JM et al: Arthroscopic debridement of the arthritic knee. Clin Orthop 1990 Apr(253):197–202

* Blau SP: The synovial fluid. Orthop Clin North Am 1979 Jan;10(1):21–35

Charcot JM: Sur quelques arthropathies qui paraissent d'ependre d'une lesion du cerveau ou de la moelle épiniere. Arch Physiol Norm Pathol 1868;1:161

** Coventry MB: Osteotomy about the knee for degenerative and rheumatoid arthritis. J Bone Joint Surg [Am] 1973 Jan;55(1):23–48

Dieppe PA, Alexander GJ, Jones HE et al: Pyrophosphate arthropathy: a clinical and radiological study of 105 cases. Ann Rheum Dis 1982 Aug;41(4):371–6

* Ewald FC: The Knee Society total knee arthroplasty roentgenographic evaluation and scoring system. Clin Orthop 1989 Nov;(248):9–12

* Fletcher MR, Scott JT: Chronic monarticular synovitis. Diagnostic and prognostic features. Ann Rheum Dis 1975 Apr;34(2):171–6

** Gunston FH: Polycentric knee arthroplasty. Prosthetic simulation of normal knee movement. J Bone Joint Surg [Br] 1971 May;53(2):272–7

Havdrup T, Hulth A, Telhag H: The subchondral bone in osteoarthritis and rheumatoid arthritis of the knee. A histological and microradiographical study. Acta Orthop Scand 1976 Jun;47(3):345–50

Insall JN: Intra-articular surgery for degenerative arthritis of the knee. A report of the work of the late K. H. Pridie. J Bone Joint Surg [Br] 1967 May;49(2):211–28

Insall JN: Total knee replacement. pp. 587–696. In Insall JN (ed): Surgery of the Knee. Churchill Livingstone, New York, 1984

Insall JN: Revision of total knee replacement. Instr Course Lect 1986;35:290–6

* Insall JN, Dorr LD, Scott RD, Scott WN: Rationale of The Knee Society clinical rating system. Clin Orthop 1989 Nov;248:13–14

Insall JN, Kelly M: The total condylar prosthesis. Clin Orthop 1986 Apr;(205):43–8

Jackson JP, Waugh W: The technique and complications of upper tibial osteotomy. A review of 226 operations. J Bone Joint Surg [Br] 1974 May;56(2):236–45

Jordan WR: Neuritic manifestations in diabetes mellitus. Arch Intern Med 1936; 57:307–366

Kaufer H, Matthews LS: Revision total knee arthroplasty: indications and contraindications. Instr Course Lect 1986;35:297–304

Klein KS, Aland CM, Kim HC et al: Long term follow-up of arthroscopic synovectomy for chronic hemophilic synovitis. Arthroscopy 1987;3(4):231–6

Landon GC, Galante JO, Maley MM: Noncemented total knee arthroplasty. Clin Orthop 1986 Apr;(205):49–57

* McKeever DC: The classic. Tibial plateau prothesis. Clin Orthop 1985 Jan–Feb;192:3–12

* Marmor L: Unicompartmental arthroplasty of the knee with a minimum ten-year follow-up period. Clin Orthop 1988 Mar;(228):171–7

Matthews LS, Goldstein SA, Malvitz TA et al: Proximal tibial osteotomy. Factors that influence the duration of satisfactory function. Clin Orthop 1988 Apr;(229):193–200

Older J, Rollinson P, Pike C: Cytological assessment of knee effusions. Arthroscopy 1988;4(3):174–8

Rittman N, Kettelkamp DB, Pryor P et al: Analysis of patterns of knee motion walking for four types of total knee implants. Clin Orthop 1981 Mar–Apr;(155):111–7

Shimizu S, Shiozawa S, Shiozawa K et al: Quantitative histologic studies on the pathogenesis of periarticular osteoporosis in rheumatoid arthritis. Arthritis Rheum 1985 Jan;28(1):25–31

Sokoloff NA: Beitrag zur Casuistik der erkrankungen der gelenke bei giomatose des ruckenmarkes (Syringomyelia). Deutsche Ztschr fur Chir 1892;34:505–548

Soudry M, Mestriner LA, Binazzi R, Insall JN: Total knee arthroplasty without patellar resurfacing. Clin Orthop 1986 Apr;(205):166–70

Thornhill TS, Scott RD: Unicompartmental total knee arthroplasty. Orthop Clin North Am 1989 Apr;20(2):245–56

* Waters RL, Perry J, Conaty P et al: The energy cost of walking with arthritis of the hip and knee. Clin Orthop 1987 Jan;(214):278–84

** Wolf AW, Benson DR, Shoji H et al: Current concepts in synovial fluid analysis. Clin Orthop 1978 July–Aug;134:261–265

** Source reference
* Reference of major interest

The Patella **10**

ANATOMY

The patella anlage appears before the 28th day of gestation. Its ossific nucleus is not roentgenographically evident until age three years in females and age four years in males. At the time of ossification, more than one center may form. The most common secondary center is located superolaterally; the incidence of bilaterality is 50 percent. The other dysplasias that have been reported are summarized in Fig. 10-1. It is important to recognize them so that they are not confused with acute fractures. The duplications are even more uncommon, with just isolated case reports in the literature (the authors have seen the duplication only in the coronal plane).

The distal pole of the patella may become elongated and develop a fragmented appearance, which should not be confused with an acute fracture. A similar fragmentation may be present at the point of insertion of the patellar ligament into the tibia. Both of these roentgenographic findings are usually bilateral and may be associated with pain and local tenderness.

The seven facets of the patella have been discussed in Chapter 1 (Fig. 10-2). The medial and lateral facets can be either concave or convex and may have different size relationships. Wiberg's three descriptions were initially thought to correlate with the incidence of patellofemoral disorders. The type I patella had equal facet sizes and was considered to be the normal. The type II had a smaller medial facet that was still concave. The type III had a smaller medial facet that was convex. The type II and III were thought to lead to increased patellofemoral pain. This anatomic finding did not prove to be reliable; however, the different facet presentations are summarized in Fig. 10-3 and are of some historical value.

The hyaline cartilage of the patellar surface is the thickest in the human body. It may range from 3 or 4 mm up to 10 or 12. This depth is thought to allow the patella to sustain pressures of three to four times the body weight. Softening of the cartilage leads to chondromalacia, and wear leads to osteoarthritis.

LIGAMENTS

The patellofemoral ligaments originate on either femoral condyle and advance anteriorly to insert into the mid portion of the medial and lateral side of the patella. They help to centralize the patella within the femoral sulcus (Fig. 10-4).

The patellar ligament originates from the distal pole of the patella and inserts into the tibial tubercle (Fig. 10-5).

Patella fragmentations

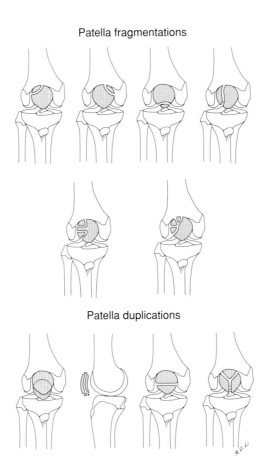

Patella duplications

Fig. 10-1. Dysplasias and duplications of the patella.

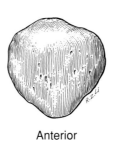

Anterior

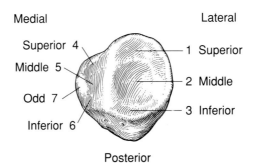

Medial   Lateral

Superior 4 ———————————— 1 Superior

Middle 5 ———————————— 2 Middle

Odd 7 ———————————— 3 Inferior

Inferior 6

Fig. 10-2. The facet anatomy of the patella.

Posterior

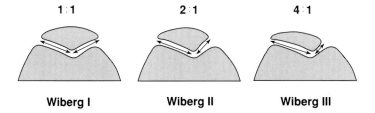

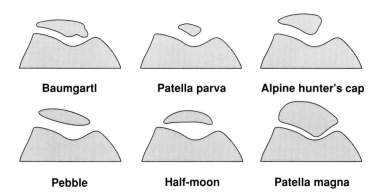

Fig. 10-3. The Wiberg patellar classifications and the variations on patellar shape.

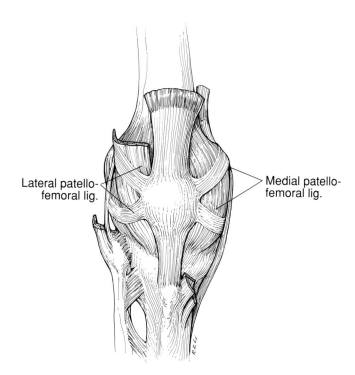

Fig. 10-4. The patellofemoral ligaments.

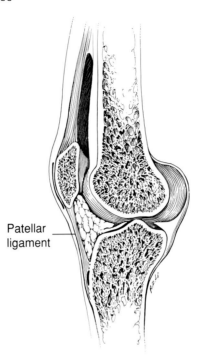

Fig. 10-5. The patellar ligament.

VASCULAR SUPPLY

The four geniculates along with the supreme geniculate and the recurrent anterior tibial arteries form a circle around the patella. Scapinelli showed that the major blood supply enters through the distal pole; thus, a transverse fracture may lead to avascular necrosis of the proximal portion. The vessels appear to enter the patella directly from the circular vasculature and not through the fat pad as was posited earlier (Fig. 10-6).

The blood supply of the patellar ligament is much less clear. The present theories favor the vessels entering from Hoffa's fat pad, which is intra-articular but extrasynovial. Actual proof for this statement is scanty.

INNERVATION

The cutaneous and muscular innervations about the patella have been discussed in Chapter 1. No nerve fibers have been found in the patella itself to account for pain syndromes; therefore, the symptoms must be explained on another basis.

BIOMECHANICS

Moments and Forces

The patella is a bony ossicle. By advancing the moment arm of the quadriceps mechanism anteriorly from the center of rotation, it increases the mechanical

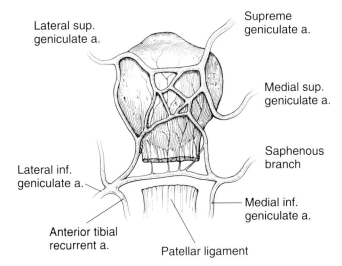

Lateral sup. geniculate a.

Supreme geniculate a.

Medial sup. geniculate a.

Saphenous branch

Lateral inf. geniculate a.

Medial inf. geniculate a.

Anterior tibial recurrent a.

Patellar ligament

Fig. 10-6. The vascular supply of the patella.

advantage of the muscle group (Fig. 10-7). The same forces created by the quadriceps mechanism create a joint reaction force across the patellar surface. The quadriceps must increase its force as the knee flexes in the weight-bearing position to overcome the moment created by the body weight. Since stress is defined as force divided by the area over which the force is applied, increased force increases the stress and increased area will decrease the stress. The increased patellofemoral contact with flexion dissipates the joint reactive force over a greater area (Fig. 10-8); however, the force can still exceed three to four times body weight with normal stair climbing. Thus, the surface of the patella must be prepared to sustain forces in the realm of *500 pounds per square inch*. This force extreme may explain why the hyaline cartilage is sometimes a full centimeter in thickness across the median ridge.

Tracking

Patellar tracking is subject to bony anatomy, lower limb alignment, muscular forces, and ligament balance. There is a natural tendency for the patella to track laterally as the knee enters the terminal 30 degrees of extension. This is very commonly seen on the Merchant skyline view (Fig. 10-9).

The lateral femoral condyle is more anterior than the medial at the superior aspect of the sulcus (Fig. 10-10). This prominence tends to oppose lateral subluxation of the patella. As flexion proceeds, the patella centralizes in the femoral groove because of the increased area of contact and the greater conformity of the two surfaces.

Lower limb alignment must take into account the femoral neck anteversion, Q angle, and tibial torsion. High anteversion with increased external torsion maximizes the Q angle and the possibilities of lateral subluxation. The patella is divided between two opposite rotations (Fig. 10-11A). High femoral neck retroversion in combination with internal tibial torsion decreases the Q angle and causes the patella to track centrally in the femoral sulcus (Fig. 10-11B).

The quadriceps mechanism also contributes to the patellar imbalance. The medialis is overwhelmed by the rectus, intermedius, and lateralis pull. Secondly, the overall vector of force is aligned with the shaft of the femur (i.e.,

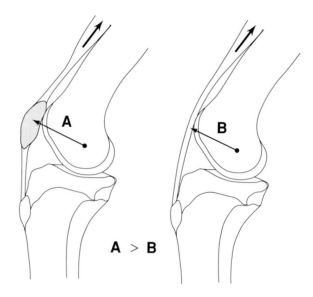

Fig. 10-7. The moment arm of the quadriceps mechanism is enhanced by the presence of the patella.

A > B

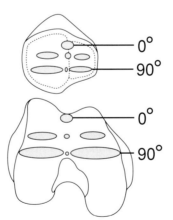

Fig. 10-8. Patellofemoral surface contact increases with flexion and spreads medially and laterally.

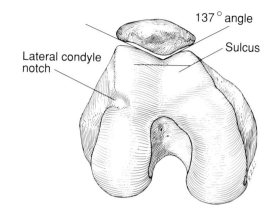

137° angle

Sulcus

Lateral condyle
notch

Fig. 10-9. The sulcus of the femur.

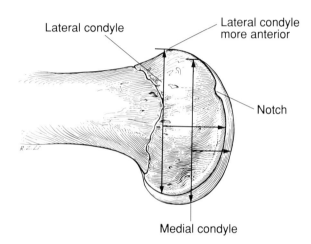

Lateral condyle

Lateral condyle
more anterior

Notch

Medial condyle

Fig. 10-10. Lateral view of the distal femur showing the anterior position of the lateral condyle and the larger size of the medial condyle.

with the anatomic axis) and not with the mechanical axis. This leads to a valgus force, away from the midline, encouraging subluxation (Fig. 10-12).

The patellofemoral ligaments help to centralize the patella, but there is some question whether the lateral ligaments are slightly tighter and shorter than the medial; this factor again favors subluxation.

Thus, a high lateral femoral condyle, low femoral neck anteversion, and internal tibial torsion are factors favoring patellar stability; however, these factors are commonly overwhelmed by the remaining anatomy.

CLINICAL ENTITIES

Symptoms of Patellofemoral Disorders

The patellofemoral joint can lead to only two symptoms: pain or instability.

Anterior knee pain, aggravated by kneeling, stair climbing, and prolonged sitting with the knee flexed is a symptom of the patellofemoral joint. On

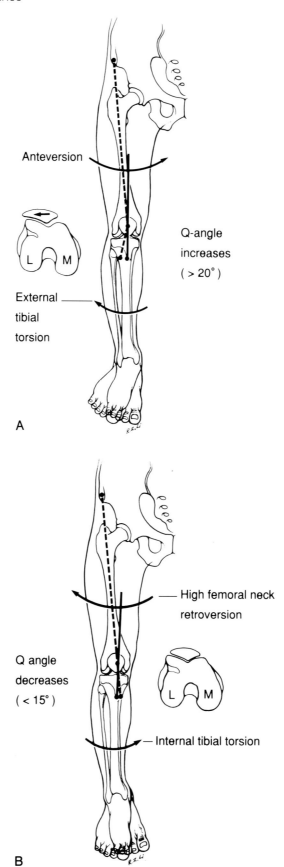

Anteversion

L   M

External
tibial
torsion

Q-angle
increases
(> 20°)

A

High femoral neck
retroversion

Q angle
decreases
(< 15°)

L   M

Internal tibial torsion

B

Fig. 10-11. (A) High femoral neck anteversion with external tibial torsion increases the Q angle leading to lateral subluxation of the patella. (B) Femoral neck retroversion in combination with internal tibial torsion decreases the Q angle and centralizes the patella.

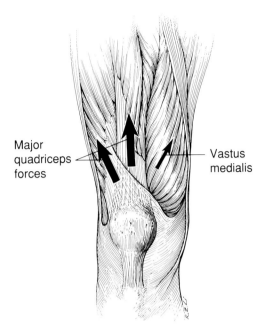

Major
quadriceps
forces

Vastus
medialis

Fig. 10-12. The quadriceps mecha-nism favors lateral distraction of the patella.

occasion, the pain can radiate or be referred to the popliteal fossa. It is seldom a global discomfort and does not involve tibiofemoral discomfort.

Dislocations or subluxations of the patella can lead to instability of the knee joint. The patient may notice the patella dislocated laterally or may relate increased instability with stair climbing. Rarely, the patella may dislocate vertically or in flexion. Then, the presentation does not include the typical lateral positioning of the patella.

With a thorough history, followed by the physical and roentgenographic examinations, it should be possible to decide whether the patellofemoral joint is the major problem. On occasion there may still be some element of clinical confusion. This can be approached with exercises and a cutout brace directed to the patellofemoral joint. If clinical improvement occurs, then the diagnosis is correct; otherwise, other areas of the knee must be implicated. It is obviously important to clarify the etiology of the discomfort before suggesting surgical intervention. Exploratory surgery of the knee is seldom acceptable.

PATELLOFEMORAL DISORDERS

Children

Patients under the age of twelve seldom present with significant patellofemoral pain without a history of trauma; however, because there are multiple dysplasias of the patella, it may sometimes become very difficult to determine if an abnormal roentgenographic appearance is the pathologic cause of the child's symptoms. Thus, it is imperative that the examiner be familiar with the skeletal aberrancies.

The most common discrepancies occur at the supralateral aspect (secondary ossification center) of the patella, at the inferior pole (particulate irregularity, Sinding-Larsen-Johansson disease), and at the tibial tubercle area (fragmentation of the tibial apophysis, Osgood-Schlatter's disease). These sites are often demonstrably tender on physical examination from inflammatory reaction. However, they do not represent areas of fracture or acute bone injury (Fig. 10-13).

Fractures of the patella are rare in the youth; however, dislocations or subluxations are often seen. The patella may dislocate because of trauma or congenital anomaly. The traumatic dislocation is treated with immobilization and exercises unless there is an associated fracture. The medial patellar facet or the lateral femoral condyle may be injured during the dislocation, leading to an intra-articular loose body requiring excision (Fig. 10-14). The congenital dislocation is caused by a flattened femoral sulcus with an atrophic patella that often articulates with a separate surface on the lateral side of the lateral femoral condyle (Fig. 10-15). The patella loses its right of domain on the femoral sulcus and commonly requires surgical realignment to stabilize the anatomy.

Adults

The primary disease of the patellofemoral joint is chondromalacia. Literally translated, this means softening of the hyaline cartilage. There are grades of involvement from mere softening, to fissures, "crabmeat changes," and, finally, to denudation down to the subchondral bone. The final stage is really one of osteoarthritis.

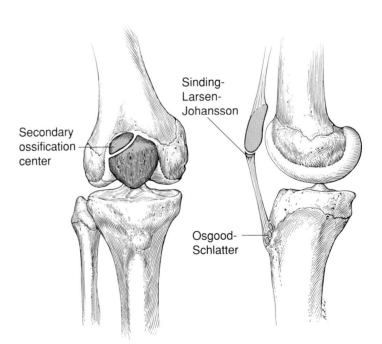

Fig. 10-13. The secondary patellar ossification center, distal pole fragmentation (Sinding-Larsen-Johansson), and tibial tubercle fragmentation (Osgood-Schlatter's) should not be mistaken for acute injuries.

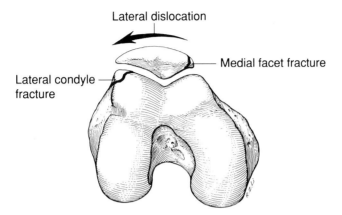

Fig. 10-14. Medial patellar facet and lateral femoral condyle fractures may be seen with patellar dislocation.

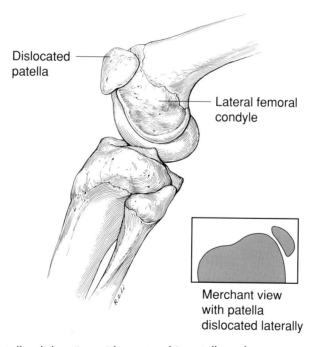

Fig. 10-15. Congenital patellar dislocation with an atrophic patella and an accessory lateral femoral condyle facet.

The stages of chondromalacia described by Bentley, Radin, and Outerbridge are often quoted to describe the extent of involvement of the patellar surface. Outerbridge's four stages are illustrated in Fig. 10-16. The pathologic changes are located in a horizontal zone across the patellar facets, with the primary area on the medial facet, the secondary on the lateral, and a lesser area between the two facets on the median ridge.

The patient presents with anterior knee pain occasionally radiating to the popliteal space.

There are four main schools of thought concerning the etiology of the pain. Some believe that malalignment of the patella explains the disease. Some believe that increased pressure develops in the joint beneath the lateral facet. Some believe that muscle dysplasia of the quadriceps group leads to irregular tracking. Some believe that there is a biochemical explanation: mechanical injury to the cartilage surface and then splitting of the proteoglycans with collagen degradation.

The treatment is often biased by one's explanation for the discomfort. The malalignment group rely upon exercises or realignment surgeries. The excess lateral pressure group rely upon lateral release of the patella to decrease the pressure. The dysplasia group tries exercises or proximal realignment, and the biochemical group uses prostaglandin synthetase inhibitors (such as aspirin or indomethacin) or non-steroidal anti-inflammatory drugs. The inhibitors are used to stop the splitting of the proteoglycans and intercept the on-going damage. The anti-inflammatory medications are an attempt to decrease the reaction after the damage has occurred.

The authors believe that the first approach to this disorder should include exercises and some form of a cutout brace to help support the patella through the range of motion. Medications have not been very successful.

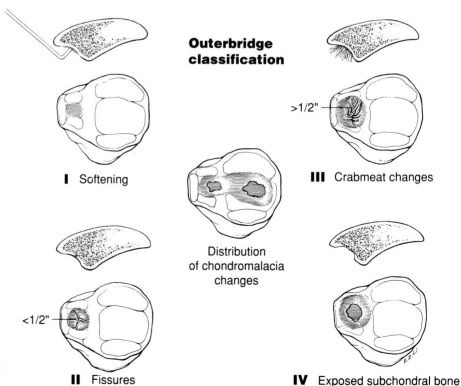

Outerbridge classification

I Softening

II Fissures

Distribution of chondromalacia changes

III Crabmeat changes

IV Exposed subchondral bone

Fig. 10-16. The chondromalacia stages according to Outerbridge.

**Table 10-1. Surgery for
Patellofemoral Disease**

Realignment	Proximal (Insall)
	Lateral release
	Distal (Elmslie-Trillat,
	    Hauser, Roux-
	    Goldthwait)

Arthroplasty	Chondroplasty (surface
	    debridement, abrasion,
	    drilling)
	Patellar resurfacing (In-
	    sall, McKeever)
	Patellofemoral replace-
	    ment

Decompression	Lateral release Maquet
Ablation	Patellectomy

Surgical intervention is indicated only in the recalcitrant case that has failed all conservative techniques. There are many surgical approaches to chondromalacia. The procedures can be grouped according to those that realign the patella (proximal, distal, or lateral release), those that try to change the surface (chondroplasty, patellar resurfacing, patellofemoral replacement), those that try to decrease the pressures (Maquet, lateral release), and those that eliminate the surface (patellectomy) (Table 10-1).

Osteoarthritis of the patellofemoral joint presents with symptoms similar to chondromalacia; however, the surface involvement is more advanced with subchondral bone exposed, and the prognosis is not as good.

Patellar dislocation in the adult is usually associated with some form of trauma and does not commonly include congenital anomalies, which lead to dislocation earlier in life. Initial dislocation is best treated with immobilization unless there is an associated medial patellar facet or lateral femoral condyle fracture. The latter problems require some form of surgical intervention to remove the loose fracture fragments.

If dislocations continue after appropriate conservative measures, then surgical realignment becomes necessary. The proximal or distal aspect of the extensor mechanism can be corrected with fairly reliable results.

Fractures, tumors, and dysplasias of the patellar surface are discussed in other areas of this book.

SUGGESTED READINGS

Ackroyd CE, Polyzoides AJ: Patellectomy for osteoarthritis. A study of eighty-one patients followed from two to twenty-two years. J Bone Joint Surg [Br] 1978 Aug;60-B(3):353 – 7

*Aglietti P, Insall JN, Cerulli G: Patellar pain and incongruence. I: Measurements of incongruence. Clin Orthop 1983 Jun;(176):217 – 24

Aglietti P, Insall JN, Walker PS, Trent P: A new patella prosthesis. Design and application. Clin Orthop 1975;107:175 – 187

** Source reference
* Reference of major interest

Batten J, Menelaus MB: Fragmentation of the proximal pole of the patella. Another manifestation of juvenile traction osteochondritis? J Bone Joint Surg [Br] 1985 Mar;67(2):249–51

**Bentley G: Articular cartilage changes in chondromalacia patellae. J Bone Joint Surg [Br] 1985 Nov;67(5):769–74

Blazina ME, Fox JM, Del Pizzo W et al: Patellofemoral replacement. Clin Orthop 1979 Oct;(144):98–102

Cash JD, Hughston JC: Treatment of acute patellar dislocation. Am J Sports Med 1988 May–Jun;16(3):244–9

**Chrisman OD, Ladenbauer-Bellis IM, Fulkerson JP: The osteoarthritic cascade and associated drug actions. Osteoarthritis Symposium Suppl Arthritis Rheum 1981;145

Chrisman OD, Snook GA, Wilson TC: The protective effect of aspirin against degradation of human cartilage. Clin Orthop 1972;84:193–206

Cox JS: An evaluation of the Elmslie-Trillat procedure for management of patellar dislocations and subluxations: A preliminary report. Am J Sports Med 1976;4:72–77

Dandy DJ, Griffiths D: Lateral release for recurrent dislocation of the patella. J Bone Joint Surg [Br] 1989 Jan;71(1):121–5

Enriquez J, Quiles M, Torres C: A unique case of dysplasia epiphysealis hemimelica of the patella. Clin Orthop 1981 Oct;(160):168–71

Ferretti A, Ippolito E, Mariani P, Puddu G: Jumper's knee. Am J Sports Med 1983 Mar–Apr;11(2):58–62

*Ficat RP, Philippe J, Hungerford DS: Chondromalacia patellae: a system of classification. Clin Orthop 1979 Oct;(144):55–62

Gasco J, Del Pino JM, Gomar-Sancho F: Double patella. A case of duplication in the coronal plane. J Bone Joint Surg [Br] 1987 Aug;69(4):602–3

Desai SS, Patel MR, Michelli LJ et al: Osteochondritis dissecans of the patella.

Hauser EDW: Total tendon transplant for slipping patella. Surg Gynec Obstet 1938;66:199–214

**Insall J: Current concepts review: patellar pain. J Bone Joint Surg [Am] 1982 Jan;64-A(1):147–52

Insall JN: Patella pain syndromes and chondromalacia patellae. Instr Course Lect 1981;30:342–56

Insall JN, Aglietti P, Tria AJ Jr: Patellar pain and incongruence. II: Clinical application. Clin Orthop 1983 Jun;(176):225–32

Jakobsen J, Christensen KS, Rasmussen OS: Patellectomy — a 20-year follow-up. Acta Orthop Scand 1985 Oct;56(5):430–2

Jerosch JG, Castro WH, Jantea C: Stress fracture of the patella. Am J Sports Med 1989 Jul–Aug;17(4):579–80

**Kaufer H: Patellar biomechanics. Clin Orthop 1979 Oct;(144):51–4

Kelly MA, Insall JN: Patellectomy. Orthop Clin North Am 1986 Apr;17(2):289–95

Levine J: A new brace for chondromalacia patella and kindred. Am J Sports Med 1978;6:137–139

Linclau L, Dokter G: Iatrogenic patella "baja". Acta Orthop Belg 1984 Jan–Feb;50(1):75–80

McKeever DC: Patellar prosthesis. J Bone Joint Surg 1955;37:1074–1084

McManus F, Rang M, Heslin DJ: Acute dislocation of the patella in children. The natural history. Clin Orthop 1979 Mar–Apr;(139):88–91

**Maquet P: Mechanics and osteoarthritis of the patellofemoral joint. Clin Orthop 1979 Oct;(144):70–3

Murakami Y: Intra-articular dislocation of the patella. A case report. Clin Orthop 1982 Nov–Dec;(171):137–9

Nottage WM, Sprague NF 3d, Auerbach BJ, Shahriaree H: The medial patellar plica syndrome. Am J Sports Med 1983 Jul–Aug;11(4):211–4

Ogden JA, Southwick WO: Osgood-Schlatter's disease and tibial tuberosity development. Clin Orthop 1976;116:180–189

Olsen EB, Trier K, Moller H: Glycosaminoglycans in patellar cartilage. Acta Orthop Scand 1989 Feb;60(1):23–5

Osgood RB: Lesions of the tibial tubercle occurring during adolescence. Boston Med Surg J 1903;148:114–117

Palumbo PM: Dynamic patellar brace: a new orthosis in the management of patellofemoral disorders. Am J Sports Med 1981;9:45–49

Peeples RE, Margo MK: Function after patellectomy. Clin Orthop 1978 May;(132):180–6

*Radin EL: A rational approach to the treatment of patellofemoral pain. Clin Orthop 1979 Oct;(144):107–9

*Reider B, Marshall JL, Warren RF: Clinical characteristics of patellar disorders in young athletes. Am J Sports Med 1981 Jul–Aug;9(4):270–4

Roux C: The classic. Recurrent dislocation of the patella: operative treatment. Clin Orthop 1979 Oct;(144):4–8

Sandow MJ, Goodfellow JW: The natural history of anterior knee pain in adolescents. J Bone Joint Surg [Br] 1985 Jan;67(1):36–8

Scapinelli R: Blood supply of the human patella. Its relation to ischemic necrosis after fracture. J Bone Joint Surg [Br] 1967;49:563–570

Scuderi G, Scharf SC, Meltzer L et al: Evaluation of patella viability after disruption of the arterial circulation. Am J Sports Med 1987 Sep–Oct;15(5):490–3

Sinding-Larsen MF: A hitherto unknown affection of the patella in children. Acta Radiol 1921;1:171–173

Sutton FS Jr, Thompson CH, Lipke J, Kettelkamp DB: The effect of patellectomy on knee function. J Bone Joint Surg [Am] 1976 Jun;58(4):537–40

van Holsbeeck M, Vandamme B, Marchal G et al: Dorsal defect of the patella: concept of its origin and relationship with bipartite and multipartite patella. Skeletal Radiol 1987;16(4):304–11

Worrell RV: Prosthetic resurfacing of the patella. Clin Orthop 1979 Oct;(144):91–7

Worrell RV: A comparison of patellectomy with prosthetic replacement of the patella. Clin Orthop 1975 Sep;(111):284–9

Zeier FG, Dissanayake C: Congenital dislocation of the patella. Clin Orthop 1980 May;(148):140–6

Congenital and Developmental Anomalies

11

Congenital and developmental deformities about the knee are uncommon; nevertheless one must be familiar with them to know which anomalies can be observed and which require prompt and aggressive therapy.

The deformities in this section will be presented according to the anatomic area involved.

THE PATELLOFEMORAL JOINT

The patella can present with two or more *ossification centers* and also can show *duplications.* These entities seldom require intervention but often can be confused with fractures of the patella (Fig. 11-1).

There are reported cases of *absence of the patella.* This is sometimes associated with other anomalies as in nail–patella syndrome (absent patella, dysplastic nails, dislocated radial heads, and iliac horns). The knee has a flattened anterior surface. If the quadriceps mechanism is intact, no intervention is necessary and exercises are instituted. If the mechanism is deficient, the hamstrings can be transferred anteriorly to assist with knee extension.

Congenital dislocation of the patella is usually associated with a hypoplastic patella that is high riding (patella alta) and tracks on the lateral wall of the lateral femoral condyle, where a secondary facet develops (Fig. 11-2). It is often associated with other anomalies of the musculoskeletal system. The deformity is present at birth but is usually overlooked because the knee is not particularly deformed; roentgenograms are not helpful because the patella is not ossified at birth. The knee is held in the flexed position with the tibia externally rotated. If this is allowed to persist, the child will eventually walk with a knee flexion contracture to avoid the pain associated with full extension.

The less extreme form of deformity is the *dislocating patella.* The patella is located anatomically in the central area of the femoral sulcus; however, because the sulcus is flattened (often at an angle of 160 to 180 degrees), the patella can readily slip out of the groove and dislocate laterally. When this occurs, there is an associated click, which is painful, sometimes audible, and brings the entity to the attention of the child and the parents.

Treatment of congenital dislocation of the patella and recurrent dislocation most commonly requires surgical intervention because neither entity responds well to conservative measures. The complete dislocation is ap-

Patella fragmentations

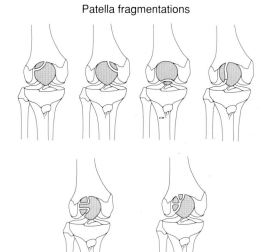

Patella duplications

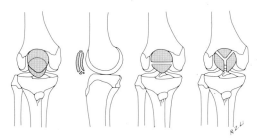

Fig. 11-1. The patellar dysplasias and duplications.

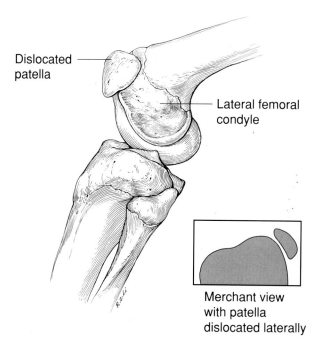

Fig. 11-2. Congenital dislocation of the patella with the patella dislocated laterally and a new facet on the lateral side of the lateral femoral condyle.

proached with a realignment of the proximal mechanism (lateral release and medial reefing). The dislocating patella can sometimes be treated with a release of the lateral capsule alone. The prognosis is good if the surface of the patella is not damaged either by the dislocations or the surgical intervention.

THE TIBIOFEMORAL JOINT

Hyperextension of the knee is a continuum from simple congenital recurvatum to subluxation and then to dislocation (Fig. 11-3). In the newborn, *recurvatum* has a clinical appearance (Fig. 11-4) similar to the other two entities, but the roentgenogram illustrates good contact of the distal femur and the proximal tibia. There is more passive flexion in recurvatum, and the knee responds to serial casting with increasing flexion.

Congenital subluxation of the tibiofemoral joint must be differentiated from *congenital dislocation* because the treatment is not the same. Congenital subluxation will show some contact of the femur with the tibia. It usually responds to manipulations and serial castings.

Congenital dislocation is equally common in both sexes and may be unilateral or bilateral. The roentgenogram shows the femoral condyles posterior to the tibia. Treatment should begin with traction followed by castings if the traction therapy is successful. If traction is not successful, open reduction should be considered.

Angular deformities of the tibiofemoral joint may be caused by the femur or the tibia. Salenius and Vankka examined the roentgenograms of pediatric patients and established normal measurements for the tibiofemoral angle. Initially, the infant has a varus knee, which converts to valgus at the age of two years. The valgus then continues to increase to approximately 15 degrees at the age of three to four years. After this age the valgus decreases slightly to the adult angulation of 5 to 10 degrees (Fig. 11-5).

On occasion, the *valgus* may be excessive. If this persists into the early teen years, some authors recommend medial femoral epiphyseal stapling if there is no significant response to bracing.

Varus deformity is usually caused by abnormality in the proximal tibia (*tibia vara* or *Blount's disease*). Langenskiold described six progressive stages of the disease with increasing age (Fig. 11-6). The stages progress from simple medial tibial fragmentation to a depression with a bone bridge from the epiphysis across to the tibial metaphysis. As the severity increases, conservative measures become less effective and surgical intervention is often necessary in the stage V and VI deformities.

In evaluating the varus knee, one should also include physiologic bowing of the tibia, Rickets, multiple enchondromatosis (Ollier's disease), trauma, and congenital tibial bowing.

INTRA-ARTICULAR ANOMALIES

The *discoid meniscus* is a circular fibrocartilage that occurs more commonly on the lateral side of the knee. The etiology is controversial. Some authors believe that the circular meniscus is a result of an arrest of development in utero; others believe that this lesion is acquired from a shortening of the ligament of Wrisberg that causes the meniscus to ride more posteriorly, with deformation of the meniscus into a discoid appearance. When the discoid meniscus presents with a tear requiring operative intervention, the initial approach is to convert the disc into a more typical C shape if this is surgically possible.

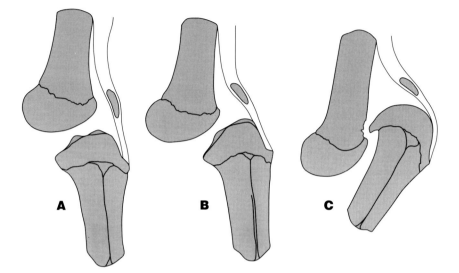

Fig. 11-3. Mild knee subluxation (A) shows some changes on the articular femorotibial surfaces, with mild anterior displacement of the tibia. These changes progress (B) and ultimately lead to complete dislocation (C).

A   B   C

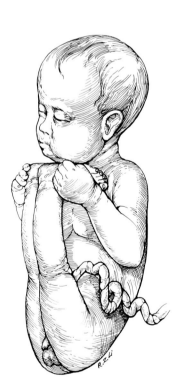

Fig. 11-4. The clinical picture of the newborn infant with congenital subluxation or dislocation of the knee.

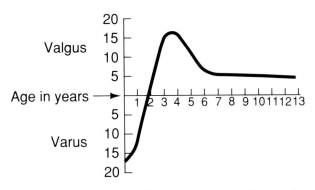

Fig. 11-5. Graph of the tibiofemoral angle with growth.

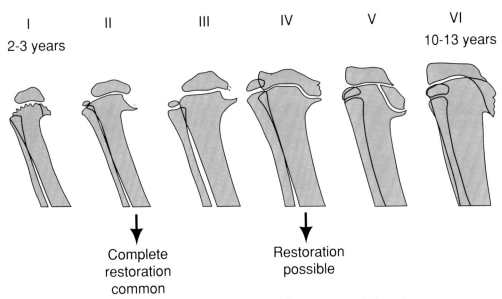

Fig. 11-6. Langenskiold's description of the six stages of Blount's disease.

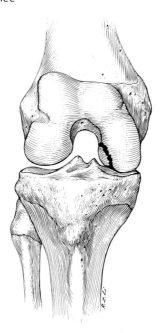

Fig. 11-7. Osteochondritis dissecans in the typical location on the
lateral wall of the medial femoral
condyle.

Osteochondritis dissecans is a lesion of the distal femur commonly on the
lateral wall of the medial femoral condyle (Fig. 11-7). It is most probably
caused by some form of vascular insult to the bone resulting in loosening of
the overlying hyaline cartilage with subchondral bone. Some schools believe
that the lesion is caused by a direct blow to the area by the tibial spines. The
typical age group is 10 to 20 years. The patient presents with localized pain
and tenderness over the site of involvement. The initial treatment is observation because the large majority of the lesions disappear after the growth
plates close. If the lesion persists or becomes loose, it can be removed.
Occasionally, the lesion may be larger and extend onto the articular surface
of the medial femoral condyle. In this case some authors advise pinning the
fragment back into position and possibly bone grafting it.

There are isolated reports of *absence of the anterior cruciate ligament.* This
abnormality is usually associated with congenital deformities of the femur or
with congenital knee dislocation. Johansson indicates that a shallow intercondylar femoral notch may be consistent with cruciate ligament absence
and believes that this roentgenographic finding may help in making the
diagnosis.

SOFT TISSUE ABNORMALITIES

Quadriceps fibrosis is a separate entity from the contracture associated with
congenital dislocation of the knee. It typically presents in the age group from
1 to 7 years with decreasing ability to flex the knee. It is often associated with
multiple injections into the quadriceps area and does not respond well to
conservative measures. Operative intervention is often successful with
lengthening of the mechanism and casting in flexion.

The *popliteal cyst* in children develops from the semimembranous bursa
beneath the medial head of the gastrocnemius muscle or directly from the
joint. Once the diagnosis has been confirmed by MRI or ultrasound, the cyst
can be followed without surgical intervention as long as it does not continue
to increase in size.

SUGGESTED READINGS

**Aichroth P: Osteochondritis dissecans of the knee. A clinical survey. J Bone Joint Surg [Br] 1971 Aug;53(3):440–7

Barrett GR, Tomasin JD: Bilateral congenital absence of the anterior cruciate ligament. Orthopedics 1988 Mar;11(3):431–4

Bell MJ, Atkins RM, Sharrard WJ: Irreducible congenital dislocation of the knee. Aetiology and management. J Bone Joint Surg [Br] 1987 May;69(3):403–6

*Carlson DH, O'Connor J: Congenital dislocation of the knee. Am J Roentgenol 1976 Sep;127(3):465–8

Chiu SS, Furuya K, Arai T et al: Congenital contracture of the quadriceps muscle. Four case reports in identical twins. J Bone Joint Surg [Am] 1974 Jul;56(5):1054–8

**Ferris B, Aichroth P: The treatment of congenital knee dislocation. A review of nineteen knees. Clin Orthop 1987 Mar;(216):135–40

Ferris BD, Jackson AM: Congenital snapping knee. Habitual anterior subluxation of the tibia in extension. J Bone Joint Surg [Br] 1990 May;72(3):453–6

*Ferrone JD Jr: Congenital deformities about the knee. Orthop Clin North Am 1976 Apr;7(2):323–30

Green JP, Waugh W, Wood H: Congenital lateral dislocation of the patella. J Bone Joint Surg [Br] 1968 May;50(2):285–9

Jacobsen K, Vopalecky F: Congenital dislocation of the knee. Acta Orthop Scand 1985 Feb;56(1):1–7

Johansson E, Aparisi T: Congenital absence of the cruciate ligaments: a case report and review of the literature. Clin Orthop 1982 Jan–Feb;(162):108–11

Johansson E, Aparisi T: Missing cruciate ligament in congenital short femur. J Bone Joint Surg [Am] 1983 Oct;65(8):1109–15

Johnson E, Audell R, Oppenheim WL: Congenital dislocation of the knee. J Pediatr Orthop 1987 Mar–Apr;7(2):194–200

Kaelin A, Hulin PH, Carlioz H: Congenital aplasia of the cruciate ligaments. A report of six cases. J Bone Joint Surg [Br] 1986 Nov;68(5):827–8

Kaplan EB: Discoid lateral meniscus of the knee joint: nature, mechanism, and operative treatment. J Bone Joint Surg [Am] 1957;39:77–87

Katz MP, Grogono BJ, Soper KC: The etiology and treatment of congenital dislocation of the knee. J Bone Joint Surg [Br] 1967 Feb;49(1):112–20

Langenskiold A: Tibia vara. Acta Chir 1952;103:1–22

Lloyd-Roberts GC, Thomas TG: The etiology of quadriceps contracture in children. J Bone Joint Surg [Br] 1964;46:498–517

Ross JA, Tough ICK, English IA: Congenital discoid meniscus. J Bone Joint Surg [Br] 1958;40:262–267

Ryan JR, Perrin JC, Morawa LG: Congenital synostosis of the knee. Clin Orthop 1978 Sep;(135):34–5

Salenius P, Vankka E: The development of the tibiofemoral angle in children. J Bone Joint Surg [Am] 1975;57:259–261

Seaton DG: Bilateral recurrent dislocation of the patellas in the Ehlers-Danlos syndrome. Med J Aust 1969 Apr 5;1(14):737–9

Steel HH, Kohl EJ: Multiple congenital dislocations associated with other skeletal anomalies (Larsen's syndrome) in three siblings. J Bone Joint Surg [Am] 1972 Jan;54(1):75–82

Storen H: Congenital complete dislocation of patella causing serious disability in childhood: the operative treatment. Acta Orthop Scand 1965;36(3):301–13

Thomas NP, Jackson AM, Aichroth PM: Congenital absence of the anterior cruciate ligament. A common component of knee dysplasia. J Bone Joint Surg [Br] 1985 Aug;67(4):572–5

Tolo VT: Congenital absence of the menisci and cruciate ligaments of the knee. A case report. J Bone Joint Surg [Am] 1981 Jul;63(6):1022–4

** Source reference
* Reference of major interest

Tumors 12

Tumors about the knee can be divided into primary and secondary (or metastatic) and benign and malignant. The most common is certainly the malignant metastatic tumor. This chapter, organized according to the four main types, will present an outline of the tumors about the knee, with the more common ones in the early portion of each discussion. No attempt will be made to review the therapeutic approaches because they are changing from day to day and far exceed the scope and principle of this book.

CLINICAL PRESENTATION AND EVALUATION

The patient with a tumorous condition of the knee often presents with non specific clinical findings. Pain, the most common symptom, is usually unrelieved with change of position and often occurs at night, even with rest. Swelling, an increasing mass, local temperature change, and local venous distention may be part of the clinical picture.

Physical examination is helpful if a mass or clinical effusion is detected. Inguinal adenopathy is occasionally present.

Roentgenograms of the knee should always form a standard part of the evaluation. MRI, CT scan, tomograms, arthrograms, and scintigraphic techniques are somewhat helpful. The plain films may show lytic or blastic lesions. Benign lesions are usually well marginated with cortical expansion but not erosion. Malignant lesions show cortical erosion, indistinct borders, and periosteal elevation (Codman's triangle). The other techniques help to identify the lesion and determine its full extent.

Laboratory tests are only occasionally helpful. The erythrocyte sedimentation rate or the peripheral white cell count may be non-specifically elevated. The alkaline phosphatase is elevated in osteogenic sarcoma and Paget's disease. The protein electrophoresis is positive in multiple myeloma.

Bone marrow biopsy may assist in the diagnosis of multiple myeloma, leukemia, and metabolic bone disease. Direct biopsy of the tumor itself is often necessary to confirm the diagnosis entertained after all of the other tests are completed.

PRIMARY TUMORS

Benign Tumors

The most common benign tumor about the knee is the *fibrous cortical defect*. These eccentric lesions have sclerotic borders, usually appear after the age of 2 years, and disappear as the child matures. The distal femoral metaphysis is the common location. The malignant potential is extremely small and the lesions seldom require biopsy.

Osteochondromas are common about the knee and are twice as prevalent on the femoral side versus the tibial. The typical age group is 10 to 20 years; the lesions are thought to be a portion of the growth plate that has been displaced; therefore, they stop increasing in size after the epiphyses close. Sarcomatous degeneration can occur, but it is extremely rare. Patients with multiple osteochondromas have a higher incidence of degeneration to a chondrosarcoma, with some clinical series reporting an incidence of 10 to 20 percent.

Approximately 10 percent of *osteoid osteomas* occur about the knee, with the predominance on the tibial metaphyseal side. Age is 10 to 20 years, with few if any tumors noted above the age of 40. The pain associated with the lesions often responds to salicylates. The tumors have a central nidus and often "burn out" with age. The *benign osteoblastoma* is thought to be a larger variant of the osteoid osteoma, with similar clinical behavior. The skeletal distribution is slightly different from the osteoid osteoma, with the majority of the lesions involving the spine.

Enchondromas are occasionally seen about the knee and tend to favor the femoral side. They should be considered because of the similar appearance to the bone infarct and the chondrosarcoma. There is very little age predominance. *Multiple enchondromatosis* (Ollier's disease) usually has a unilateral distribution with a higher incidence of sarcomatous degeneration.

Chondroblastomas are less common tumors in general but have a predilection for the knee. About 30 percent of all lesions occur there, with equal division between the femoral and the tibial side. The typical age is between 10 and 20 years. The tumor is radiolucent and is usually located in the epiphysis.

Both the *aneurysmal and unicameral bone cysts* occur about the knee, but in only approximately 10 percent or less of the cases. The unicameral cyst is usually in a younger population (age 4 to 10 years) while the aneurysmal cyst may be seen in ages from 10 to 20. The malignant potential is low and many of the lesions resolve without intervention.

Synovial chondromatosis is a cartilaginous metaplasia of synovium often seen in the knee. The roentgenogram demonstrates multiple flocculent calcifications about the joint. The age group is not specific but it occurs in the adult population. It has a tendency to recur after synovectomy but has almost no malignant potential.

Pigmented villonodular synovitis is a benign lesion of the synovial lining of the knee. It may be localized to one or two sessile or stalked growths, or it may be diffuse. The patients are young adults. Eighty per cent of the lesions involve the hip or knee areas. Synovectomy is the procedure of choice; the recurrence rate is quite high.

Malignant Tumors

The most common site for *giant cell tumors* is about the knee (50 percent of lesions). These radiolucent tumors are typically located in the epiphysis of the long bones and are equally common on the femoral and tibial side. The typical age is 20 to 30 years. The prognosis is proportional to the grade of the malignancy seen with each tumor (grading is from one to three).

Fifty percent of *osteogenic sarcomas* occur about the knee, with twice as many lesions on the femoral than the tibial side. Average age is 20 to 30 years. The prognosis is changing rapidly with new methods of chemotherapy and resections.

Fibrosarcoma, chondrosarcoma, malignant fibrous histiocytoma, and *juxtacortical osteogenic sarcoma,* far less common tumors, all have a tendency to occur about the knee, with an incidence from 30 to 70 percent for each individual lesion. Adamantinoma is primarily a tibial tumor and can occasionally be seen in the metaphyseal area near the knee joint. These lesions favor ages from 40 to 70 years.

SECONDARY TUMORS

Benign Tumors

These lesions are rarely seen. The brown tumor of hyperparathyroidism is probably the most common.

Malignant Tumors

Metastatic lesions are uncommon about the knee but must be considered as a possible entity. Multiple myeloma and metastases from breast, lung, prostate, thyroid, kidney, and the gastrointestinal tract are some of the common primary sources. The roentgenographic presentation may be one of a lytic or blastic nature. The age group includes an older population seldom under the age of 50 years.

DIAGNOSTIC EVALUATION

Because discomfort in the knee can be associated with the above lesions, every thorough examination should include a complete set of standard roentgenograms. Many of the lesions can be diagnosed by the roentgenogram alone. Other tumors will require special studies or a complete evaluation to rule out a primary process elsewhere in the body. With the dawn of new technologies such as MRI, there is sometimes a tendency to omit the plain roentgenograms and go directly to special studies. At the present time, this represents an error in judgment.

SUGGESTED READINGS

**Aegerter E, Kirkpatrick JA Jr: Orthopedic Diseases. WB Saunders, Philadelphia, 1975
*Aisen AM, Martel W, Braunstein EM et al: MRI and CT evaluation of primary bone and soft-tissue tumors. AJR Am J Roentgenol 1986 Apr;146(4):749–56

** Source reference
* Reference of major interest

Braidwood AS, McDougall A: Adamantinoma of the tibia. Report of two cases. J Bone Joint Surg [Br] 1974 Nov;56-B(4):735–8

*Campanacci M, Picci P, Gherlinzoni F et al: Parosteal osteosarcoma. J Bone Joint Surg [Br] 1984 May;66(3):313–21

**Dahlin DC: Bone Tumors. Charles C Thomas, Springfield, Ill, 1978

*Dahlin DC, Cupps RE, Johnson EW Jr: Giant-cell tumor: a study of 195 cases. Cancer 1970 May;25(5):1061–70

De Coster E, Van Tiggelen R, Shahabpour M et al: Osteoblastoma of the patella. Case report and review of the literature. Clin Orthop 1989 Jun;(243):216–9

deSantos LA, Murray JA, Finklestein JB et al: The radiographic spectrum of periosteal osteosarcoma. Radiology 1978 Apr;127(1):123–9

Ehara S, Khurana JS, Kattaspuram SV et al: Osteolytic lesions of the patella. AJR Am J Roentgenol 1989 Jul;153(1):103–6

Fineschi G, Schiavone Panni A: Free patellar graft for the reconstruction of juxtaarticular defects in the treatment of giant-cell tumors. Clin Orthop 1990 Jul;(256):197–204

*Goldenberg RR, Campbell CJ, Bonfiglio M: Giant-cell tumor of bone. An analysis of two hundred and eighteen cases. J Bone Joint Surg [Am] 1970 Jun;52(4):619–64

Hall RB, Robinson LH, Malawar MM, Dunham WK: Periosteal osteosarcoma. Cancer 1985 Jan 1;55(1):165–71

**Jaffe HL: Tumors and Tumorous Conditions of Bones and Joints. Lea & Febiger, Philadelphia, 1958

*Joyce MJ, Mankin HJ: Caveat arthroscopos: extra-articular lesions of bone simulating intra-articular pathology of the knee. J Bone Joint Surg [Am] 1983 Mar;65(3):289–92

Linscheid RL, Dahlin DC: Unusual lesions of the patella. J Bone Joint Surg [Am] 1966 Oct;48(7):1359–66

Marcove RC, Lyden JP, Huvos AG, Bullough PB: Giant-cell tumors treated by cryosurgery. A report of twenty-five cases. J Bone Joint Surg [Am] 1973 Dec;55(8):1633–44

McLeod RA, Beabout JW: The roentgenographic features of chondroblastoma. Am J Roentgenol Radium Ther Nucl Med 1973 Jun;118(2):464–71

McLeod RA, Dahlin DC, Beabout JW: The spectrum of osteoblastoma. Am J Roentgenol 1976 Feb;126(2):321–5

Micheli LJ, Jupiter J: Osteoid osteoma as a cause of knee pain in the young athlete: a case study. Am J Sports Med 1978 Jul–Aug;6(4):199–203

Moser RP Jr, Brockmole DM, Vinh TN et al: Chondroblastoma of the patella. Skeletal Radiol 1988;17(6):413–9

Ogden JA: Multiple hereditary osteochondromata. Report of an early case. Clin Orthop 1976 May;(116):48–60

Patel MR, Desai SS: Patellar metastases. A case report and review of the literature. Orthop Rev 1988 Jul;17(7):687–90

Picci P, Manfrini M, Zucchi V et al: Giant-cell tumor of bone in skeletally immature patients. J Bone Joint Surg [Am] 1983 Apr;65(4):486–90

Puddu G, Mariani P: Osteoid osteoma of the Gerdy's tubercle in an athlete. A case report. Am J Sports Med 1981 Jan–Feb;9(1):57–9

Springfield DS, Capanna R, Gherlinzoni F et al: Chondroblastoma. A review of seventy cases. J Bone Joint Surg [Am] 1985 Jun;67(5):748–55

Stoler B, Staple TW: Metastases to the patella. Radiology 1969 Oct;93(4):853–6

Wilson JS, Genant HK, Carlsson A, Murray WR: Patellar giant cell tumor. Am J Roentgenol 1976 Nov;127(5):856–8

Infections of the Knee **13**

Infections of the knee can be divided into those that involve the extra-articular spaces (such as the pre-patellar space), the intra-articular space, and the underlying bone. Such infections can be primary in the knee area itself or may be "metastatic" from another source in the body cavities.

Knee arthroplasty infection will be considered as a separate entity.

EXTRA-ARTICULAR INFECTION

There are spaces about the knee that can become areas of localized infection. The prepatellar bursa, pretibial bursa, and the pes anserine bursa are the common spaces. Infection in each of these areas is walled off from the knee joint itself. The offending organism is usually *Streptococcus* or *Staphylococcus aureus*. The knee presents with a localized area of erythema, swelling, and sometimes fluctuance. The erythema often resembles a cellulitis. Local treatment with moist heat and appropriate oral antibiotics is usually sufficient. Aspiration of the space for the purposes of diagnosis is seldom necessary and if undertaken must be performed with care to avoid transgressing the underlying joint space and implanting infection in the joint itself. On occasion these infections may be difficult to control and may require open drainage, or may drain spontaneously. Once this has occurred, the healing process is prolonged.

INTRA-ARTICULAR INFECTION

Primary infection of the knee joint is not common without another underlying condition (such as a compromised host or a rheumatoid patient who has undergone multiple aspirations). When joint infection is suspected, a thorough evaluation should be completed. Plain roentgenograms, a complete blood count with white cell differential, an erythrocyte sedimentation rate, and a joint aspiration should be completed. While bone scans are more helpful for infection in the osseous structures, the early flow studies may show increase to the joint and support the suspicion of infection.

The most valuable of all of the tests is certainly the aspiration performed for culture. At the same time, the fluid can be examined as outlined in Table 9-1. Septic fluid will have a turbid to purulent appearance with poor mucin clot. The sugar level will be lower than the blood serum sugar level and the cell count will be elevated to over 100,000, with the majority of the cells polymorphonuclear.

If the joint is infected without evidence of bone involvement, there are two main therapeutic approaches: multiple aspirations or operative drainage. There are many articles in the literature to support both techniques. At present, gram positive infections can sometimes be controlled with aspirations, but the knee joint must be observed closely to be sure that it is responding appropriately without extension of the infection to the bone or the overlying soft tissues. If this becomes the case, then open drainage must be performed. Gram negative infections are best controlled with operative drainage. Even with complete lavage of the joint, it is often difficult to control such infections. Both therapeutic regimens require parenteral antibiotics for a minimum of 4 to 6 weeks. The prognosis is fairly good if the infection is treated early and aggressively.

BONE INFECTION

Infection in the knee joint may involve the bone itself. The diagnosis can be confirmed by technetium, gallium and indium bone scanning techniques. All three of these tests should show increase in uptake in the underlying bone with the differential favoring the gallium and the indium scans. The erythrocyte sedimentation rate should be elevated, the peripheral white count may be mildly increased, and a bone biopsy should be positive for the offending organism. Treatment involves appropriate parenteral antibiotics with possible incision and drainage of the involved area of bone if the antibiotics fail to control the infection or a sequestrum develops.

ARTHROPLASTY INFECTION

A separate section should be devoted to the infected knee arthroplasty. This is a complex problem not only because of the joint infection but also because of the presence of a significant foreign body in the knee. The infections should be divided between the acute and the delayed.

The *acute infection* occurs within two weeks of the original surgery. One's suspicions should always be high, and the joint aspiration is the most important study. If the problem is noticed early, the joint can sometimes be saved by irrigating the arthroplasty in the operating room and treating the patient with six weeks of parenteral antibiotics; joint aspirations should be cultured after the regimen has been completed.

The *chronic* or *late infection* occurs several weeks, months, or years after the original surgery. The diagnosis is more difficult to confirm. The patient usually presents with a painful knee joint that is moderately swollen. There is seldom a significant elevation in the patient's temperature and the peripheral white cell count is seldom elevated. The erythrocyte sedimentation rate is mildly elevated and the gallium and indium scans are usually positive. Roentgenograms may show radiolucency about one or more of the components at the bone-cement interface and may also include periosteal reaction. The aspiration of the joint is usually positive. The differential diagnosis must also include a simple joint sprain with resultant effusion and a sterile prosthetic loosening.

The chronic infection must initially be controlled with prosthetic removal and thorough joint debridement. If the infection is surgically controlled before a fistulous tract develops through the skin, it is sometimes possible to reimplant the prosthesis after appropriate parenteral antibiotic therapy (minimum of 4 to 6 weeks). Once a fistula has developed, the soft tissues about the knee are significantly contaminated and successful reimplantation is highly unlikely.

Gram positive infections have a fair prognosis. Gram negative infections have a poor prognosis. Before any reimplantation is considered, one must be sure that the joint itself is sterile and that no residual infection is present.

SUGGESTED READINGS

*Bengtson S, Blomgren G, Knutson K et al: Hematogenous infection after knee arthroplasty. Acta Orthop Scand 1987 Oct;58(5):529–34

**Borden LS, Gearen PF: Infected total knee arthroplasty. A protocol for management. J Arthroplasty 1987;2(1):27–36

*Brause BD: Infections associated with prosthetic joints. Clin Rheum Dis 1986 Aug;12(2):523–36

Bynum DK Jr, Nunley JA, Goldner L, Martinez S: Pyogenic arthritis: Emphasis on the need for surgical drainage of the infected joint. South Med J 1982;75:1232–1238

Freeman MA, Sudlow RA, Casewell MW, Radcliff SS: The management of infected total knee replacements. J Bone Joint Surg [Br] 1985 Nov;67(5):764–8

Friedman RJ, Friedrich LV, White RL et al: Antibiotic prophylaxis and tourniquet inflation in total knee arthroplasty. Clin Orthop 1990 Nov;(260):17–23

**Goldenberg DL, Brandt KD, Cohen AS, Cathcart ES: Treatment of septic arthritis: Comparison of needle aspiration and surgery as initial modes of joint drainage. Arthritis Rheum 1975;18:83–90

Glynn MK, Sheehan JM: An analysis of the causes of deep infection after hip and knee arthroplasties. Clin Orthop 1983 Sep;(178):202–6

Hall AJ: Late infection about a total knee prosthesis. Report of a case secondary to urinary tract infection. J Bone Joint Surg [Br] 1974 Feb;56(1):144–7

**Insall JN: Infection of total knee arthroplasty. Instr Course Lect 1986;35:319–24

Ivey M, Clark R: Arthroscopic debridement of the knee for septic arthritis. Clin Orthop 1985;199:201–206

Marmor L, Berkus D: Hematogenous infection of total knee implants. Surgery 1978 Mar;83(3):291–2

Marsh PK, Cotler JM: Management of an anaerobic infection in a prosthetic knee with long-term antibiotics alone: a case report. Clin Orthop 1981 Mar–Apr;(155):133–5

McKillop JH, McKay I, Cuthbert GF et al: Scintigraphic evaluation of the painful prosthetic joint: a comparison of gallium-67 citrate and indium-111 labelled leucocyte imaging. Clin Radiol 1984 May;35(3):239–41

Rodeheaver GT, Rukstalis D, Bono M, Bellamy W: A new model of bone infection used to evaluate the efficacy of antibiotic-impregnated polymethylmethacrylate cement. Clin Orthop 1983 Sep;(178):303–11

*Salvati EA, Robinson RP, Zeno SM et al: Infection rates after 3175 total hip and total knee replacements performed with and without a horizontal unidirectional filtered air-flow system. J Bone Joint Surg [Am] 1982 Apr;64(4):525–35

Waters P, Kasser J: Infection of the infrapatellar bursa. A report of two cases. J Bone Joint Surg [Am] 1990 Aug;72(7):1095–6

Windsor RE, Insall JN, Urs WK et al: Two-stage reimplantation for the salvage of total knee arthroplasty complicated by infection. Further follow-up and refinement of indications. J Bone Joint Surg [Am] 1990 Feb;72(2):272–8

** Source reference

* Reference of major interest

Index

Numbers followed by f *indicate figures, and those followed by* t *indicate tables.*